CAROLE MAGGIO

FACERCISE®

CAROLE MAGGIO

FACERCISE®

The Dynamic Muscle-Toning Program for
Renewed Vitality and
a More Youthful Appearance

BY CAROLE MAGGIO

WITH KYLE RODERICK

A PERIGEE BOOK

As with any exercise, the reader may wish to consult with
a physician before beginning the fitness program presented in this
book. Responsibility for any adverse affects resulting from the use
of information contained herein rests solely with the reader.

A Perigee Book
Published by The Berkley Publishing Group
200 Madison Avenue
New York, NY 10016

First edition: May 1995

Published simultaneously in Canada.

Library of Congress Cataloging-in-Publication Data
Maggio, Carole.
　　Carole Maggio facercise / Carole Maggio.—1st ed.
　　　p.　　cm.
　　ISBN 0-399-51960-2
　　1. Middle aged women—Health and hygiene. 2. Facelift. 3. Face—Care and hygiene.
4. Beauty, Personal. I. Title. II. Title: Facercise.
RA778.M26　　1995
646.7'26—dc20　　　　　　　　　　　　　　　　　　　　94-43974
　　　　　　　　　　　　　　　　　　　　　　　　　　　　　CIP

Printed in the United States of America

10　9　8　7　6　5

This book is dedicated to my dear friend, Joan Christensen. Without her unending support this book would not have been written. To my sister, Michal, who pushed me to continue to share my dream, and to Gloria, whose "vision" always inspired me to help others achieve their dreams.

CONTENTS

CAROLE MAGGIO

FACERCISE®

INTRODUCTION

All attractive women share the same beauty secret: they care enough to make the best of their unique features. Although there are few things in this world that we can control, you *can* control how well you look, if you're willing to make the effort. This book is a key to your self-improvement efforts.

I have successfully taught Facercise for more than eleven years to hundreds of clients across the United States, England, France, Brunei, Hong Kong, Singapore, Jordan, and Japan. Facercise will teach you the skills to help you recapture and maintain a younger, healthier, and more vital-looking face.

Facercise is a natural approach to reshaping your facial appearance. When devising the exercises, I consulted with plastic surgeons and other M.D.'s to ensure their safety and effectiveness. By carefully following the Facercise program, you can strengthen and develop the facial muscles so that the face is actually restructured to achieve an improved, younger look. With Facercise, you can take ten years off your face, without silicone, stitches, or surgery. All you have to do is work your facial muscles.

Just as a body builder develops his or her physique by isolating and working muscles one by one, you can accentuate or develop cheeks, lips, the eye area, and other facial features by repeating a specific exercise.

Because the muscles in the face are so small and responsive, dramatic results can be achieved quickly, sometimes in a matter of hours.

By working out the facial muscles underneath the skin, you tone and tighten up the underlying structure of your face. Performing Facercise properly also increases the blood circulation in the skin, so pale or sallow complexions become peachy-pink and glowing. The overall result is a firmly toned, rosier face: within three days, there is usually a noticeable improvement in the facial contours and complexion.

To understand the benefits that you will enjoy from Facercise, let's first consider how the face ages. We have fifty-seven facial muscles, but we rarely work most of them. As you age, muscles flatten and elongate with lack of use and the pull of gravity; sagging skin is the inevitable result. As time passes, the bone, muscle, and fat under the facial skin—and elsewhere on the body—actually diminishes, while, at the same time, the skin loses its elasticity. By now, most of us are aware that sunbathing and environmental stress cause wrinkles, but habitual facial movements—such as furrowing your brow and squinting when you're confused—can also etch lines into your skin.

Although surgery can pull the skin tight across the face and lift it up, the elements that cause wrinkles and sags still remain and ultimately prevail. In time, the same wrinkles and sags that were present before surgery reappear to varying degrees. Many people who sign on for plastic surgery eventually find themselves too gravity-stricken or age-afraid to get off the merry-go-round.

Whereas plastic surgery deals with the symptoms of aging skin, Facercise deals with some of the causes: weakened underlying muscle and constricted blood circulation in the face. While a surgical face-lift can offer visible results, it's an expensive and painful procedure with short-lived benefits. Face-lifts routinely require follow-up surgery after several years, and with each additional surgery, the face often appears more tightly stretched. Face-lifted faces can appear hard and masklike—anything but youthful.

For far less money and discomfort than plastic surgery entails, Facercise provides natural, long-term results that are much more appealing. Instead of putting your destiny in the hands of a plastic surgeon, Facercise empowers you by giving you ultimate control over your face. This program will give your looks a lift without scars or having to wear your eyebrows in the middle of your forehead, like some plastic-surgery veterans I've seen.

Facercise is not a one-time procedure but a continuing improvement program. Be patient, read the exercise instructions closely, and *practice*.

Once you've mastered the Facercise exercises, you can do them anywhere, anytime—in the car, on the phone, while you're doing housework or sitting at a computer. Do your Facercise properly and you will continue to improve your appearance every week, every month, and as the years go by. Just how youthful you grow is up to you!

1

HELP YOUR FACE!

My fascination with beauty began in, of all places, an elevator. I was fourteen years old at the time, and was standing beside my mother when a woman with a strange-looking, unnaturally tight face stepped in. I couldn't take my eyes off her. When we got off the elevator, I asked my mother, "What in the world was wrong with that woman's face?"

"She's had a face-lift, Carole," she said. "You know, they call it plastic surgery."

That woman in the elevator was someone I was determined never to look like. I instinctively felt that her face-lift had achieved the opposite effect of a beautiful face. I believe that looking as good as possible is part of living a full and happy life, but I also know there are many roads to beauty. I've always been concerned with my looks, and I have always cared very much how other women look. I love seeing a woman look her very best.

In my early twenties, I started a real estate career, got married, and had a family, but my avid interest in beauty became an active sideline activity. I read everything I could on the subject, from beauty magazines to medical books; I studied and kept files. This research into the art of skin care, with a special interest in anti-aging treatments and cosmetics, ultimately led to a career change.

Within six years, I became a licensed esthetician and opened a skin and figure salon in Monterey, California. At that time I myself was combatting two common beauty flaws: cellulite and dry, lined skin from too many years of suntanning. I knew that if I needed help with these problems, then other women probably did, too. The salon was a great success, and it afforded me the valuable experience of working with so many different women. I learned to see how a woman's face becomes a map of her habits, her emotional history, and her state of mind. And I learned how to enhance each woman's unique beauty.

In the seven years that I ran my salon, I refined my knowledge of the latest and most touted beauty treatments. I flew around the world to take classes with the foremost professionals in the field. I took training from Beverly Hills skin care experts and medical doctors to acquire rare information and expertise. Dr. Gerald Snyder taught me the hand-lift massage, a wonderful skill to master. The massage toned the skin and increased blood circulation so much that it made my clients look like they had just had a face-lift. Although this massage was extremely effective, the "face-lift" only lasted a week. Still, my clients felt wonderful and looked better as each week of treatment went by.

I used a variety of skin care regimens in the salon. At one time I was carrying items from nine different lines because I couldn't find any one that offered all the results I sought.

By the time I was thirty-six years old, the fine lines on my face were growing more visible—and more difficult to fill out. Although I performed anti-aging treatments such as lymphatic drainage and hand-lift massage in my salon, I could not perform these methods on myself. And none of my employees could do them because the techniques were too specialized. Imagine my frustration: I could work wonders for my clients but was incapable of improving my own appearance.

Around this time my husband, who is sixteen years my senior, casually mentioned that he thought I was looking my age and then some. I was devastated. But I knew he was right. The good news is that his remark made me take stock of my situation—and then my inspiration came. I realized that if I could somehow plump up the underlying structure of my face, the lines would fill out and diminish. My face would appear smoother and more toned.

I began to study the anatomy of the face and to learn how the facial muscles work. I read textbooks on the theory of exercise, and I studied and experimented until I knew how to isolate and manipulate the major muscles in my face. Slowly and carefully, I began to develop an exercise program that would "re-contour" my face the way I wanted it to look.

I worked away in secret like some kind of beauty spy, just trying to find some way to help myself. After about six weeks of "working out," one of my regular clients confronted me excitedly and said, "What are you doing to your face? You look younger." I confided that I had been creating and practicing facial exercises.

"Teach me how to work out the same way," she said. She was that impressed with the positive changes she saw in my face. I explained that I wasn't sure I could teach anyone what I'd been doing in private—after all, the exercises were something that I had been refining for myself, on myself—but I'd be happy to give her face a try.

If only I had taken a picture of this woman before we began working together. I had no idea how rapidly I could teach her to develop the muscles of her face. I devised a twenty-minute daily program for her, and to our mutual delight, her appearance changed dramatically in just five days.

Six days after we first started working together, she asked me to take a Polaroid snapshot, and the next day she brought in a photo that had been taken three years before. When we placed the photos side by side, the difference was strikingly obvious. Not only did her face look younger, well toned, and rosier, but there was a new light in her eyes. The exercises had increased circulation and oxygen flow in the muscles around her eyes, and they were sparkling. This woman sent me the first of many client letters thanking me for the great improvements that I have made in their appearances. (I've included some other testimonials at the back of the book—look for them after Chapter Six.)

I felt quite touched by the gratitude of my first Facercise client, but I reminded her, "I may have given you the tools, but you did the work. Thank yourself." And I meant it. This wonderful lady committed herself to working on her face, and she looked fantastic. She deserved to feel proud. This success with my first Facercise client led me to the conclusion that if people are willing to spend hours each week exercising their bodies, then they should be willing to give their faces a few minutes a day, too.

I was right, and word of mouth about my exercises spread quickly. After achieving similarly great improvements with clients of all ages, I acquired a professional understanding of how different faces age and how they can be revitalized by working the muscles underneath.

Through working with various women—and a few men—I learned how to raise eyebrows, shorten noses, enlarge lips, plump up cheeks, and tighten jawlines and triple chins. I also grew to see how, as the years go by, we naturally lose the fat cells in the face. Our bones shrink, and the aging face can take on a more brittle or saggy look. I even noticed—and later read medical documentation that confirmed my observation—that the nose lengthens throughout life. It never stops growing! As I saw people benefit from my facial exercises, I envisioned how every face, regardless of age, shape, or texture, could derive anti-aging benefits from a custom-designed exercise program—and thus Facercise was born! And Facercise delivered a bonus beauty treatment: the exercises proved to be great stress-relievers. Facercise would wage battle on frown lines, angry mouths, and worry lines—on two fronts!

As my Facercise business grew, I continued to research the benefits and drawbacks of cosmetic surgery. I realized that for some people, successful cosmetic surgery can rejuvenate their looks and polish their self-image and confidence. But plastic surgery may not be the answer for everyone. A face-lift stretches and pulls the skin and muscles back to the ears; it can emphasize the aging, brittle look of one's features. I'm talking about the same artificially tight look that I first saw in the lady in the elevator when I was fourteen.

I know that there are some surgeons who are masters of reconstruction and beautification. To find a good doctor always involves research, and the more research you do, the better the chances you'll find an artist-surgeon. You must start by collecting referrals from satisfied patients, then you can interview doctors and look at photographs of their work before you make any decisions.

The most enlightened doctors realize that there are important adjuncts to plastic surgery, such as customized skin care and facial exercises. Many plastic surgeons refer their patients to me because they know that Facercise can help reconstruct and reshape muscles weakened from face-lifts and other surgical modifications. When done properly, Facercise strengthens the muscles and helps maintain the beneficial looks of plastic surgery.

About 60 percent of my clients are people who have had some form of plastic surgery—an eyelift, a rhinoplasty, or a complete face-lift. Not all of these surgeries were successful, and I tell you, I can sympathize with people who are disappointed with their cosmetic surgery. You see, I survived a bad nose job that left a dent on the left side of my nose! Yet Facercise helped shorten my nose tip (it had been left too long) and fill out the dent. Now it's invisible.

Many of my clients who have had cosmetic surgery are determined not to go back for follow-up operations five to seven years down the road.

In that first year after surgery, I teach them to exercise and build up the facial muscles to prevent the need for subsequent maintenance operations. Facercise gives them good results and a sense of control over their own destinies.

While I'm not opposed to cosmetic surgery, I think it's worth noting that there is always an element of risk involved. Even the greatest surgeons can fail to deliver the results they promise. Health, age, and skin elasticity all influence how the face will respond to surgery. There are so many variables to be considered, whereas with facial exercises, the process is risk-free and results are predictably beneficial. By learning how to pump your facial muscles, you will nourish every cell in your face with life-giving blood.

A natural alternative to surgical intervention, Facercise provides a gentle and ever-renewable way for an individual to triumph over his or her genetic destiny. (Many of my clients come to me when their mouths start to look like their mothers'!) Facercise helps reinvent a younger, more relaxed-looking face. After a single session with one of my honest-to-God royal clients, she told me, "I've been looking for someone like you for ten years! Now there's no need to resort to a face-lift!"

My clients (civilians and monarchs alike!) range in age from twenty to eighty-seven. My eighty-seven-year-old is an energetic lady who loves tap dancing and now looks as young as she feels, since her Facercise training. Many of my younger clients are already veterans of unsuccessful plastic surgeries, and the older of them enjoy a vital shot of self-esteem from "lifting" their faces with Facercise. Experience has shown me that you're never really too old—or too young—to start Facercise.

Some of my most interesting clients are people who use Facercise to help overcome physiological damage sustained from paralyzing illnesses or disfiguring car accidents. I once trained a man in his fifties who had been stricken decades before with Bell's Palsy, a condition which had paralyzed one side of his face and partially closed an eye. From the very first day of our sessions, he threw himself into his exercises, despite his disability. By the second afternoon, he had started regaining feeling in his formerly paralyzed facial muscles. His eyes welled with tears.

"Carole," he said, his voice breaking with emotion, "After thirty-five years I have feeling in my face—the numbness is gone. Thank you for helping me in a way that no doctor ever has."

It intrigues me whenever I read or hear an interview with a dermatologist or a plastic surgeon on the subject of facial exercises. Those who know nothing about it will make statements to the effect that there is no scientific proof that facial exercises are effective in recontouring the face. Yet some of the world's leading medical authorities have gone on record in favor of facial exercises.

According to Wilma Bergfeld, M.D., the president of the American Academy of Dermatology, "Exercising facial muscles in a reasonable fashion certainly can improve the general appearance of the skin's surface without harming it in any way." Many physicians also see the therapeutic value of Facercise. Lawrence Birnbaum, M.D., a Beverly Hills plastic surgeon, says, "The exercises as taught by Ms. Maggio are extremely beneficial to both pre- and post-operative cosmetic surgery patients. They can also help anyone else lift sagging facial skin via building up the fifty-seven facial muscles."

After I had spent a few years teaching Facercise in the United States, word of mouth about the exercises went global and my business blossomed all over the world. I've taught international celebrities and business leaders you read about in magazines, and I've been summoned by movie stars to film sets the day they're shooting close-ups. My career highlights include giving Facercise seminars for beauty professionals at the University of London and at the Les Nouvelles Esthetiques Congresses in France and England. In 1994 I addressed the Beauty and Health Conference in Hong Kong, and a few months later the British women's magazine *Harpers & Queen* invited me to speak at a glamorous charity benefit sponsored by the Italian fashion house Emporio Armani.

I have been teaching Facercise for more than ten years now, and I am continually refining, expanding, and updating the exercises. Although I first started doing the exercises with women, today about a quarter of my clients are men. My male clients include Hollywood actors, business executives, British rock stars, and Middle Eastern royalty.

Although I'm proud of the way Facercise is tailored to enhance and maintain individual facial features, I also want to stress that you don't have to do the whole twenty-minute program in one sitting. It's a flexible, adaptable routine; the exercises can be easily merged into your day. For example, you can do your eye exercises while talking on the phone or while you wait to pick up your kids at the bus stop. Do your nose exercises while you read during your lunch hour. I have even tailored all of the exercises so that they can be done while driving the car.

Facercise is just about the most user-friendly health and beauty regimen ever invented. Consider this book a personal trainer for your face, and your mirror will provide progress reports.

I take photographs of new clients before they begin the program and then a few days later. I have hundreds of these photos I've collected over the years. The camera never lies. Changes are visible in a photograph after just a few days of doing Facercise twenty minutes a day. Those who devote twenty minutes a day to the exercises for at least five days a week often see results greater than ever hoped for outside of surgery. The pictures are proof positive. (If you just can't wait any longer, you'll find some in Chapter Three.)

I want my clients to understand how Facercise will help them in ways that plastic surgery cannot. That's why I talk straight to them about the perils and possibilities of aging faces. Although gravity pulls your face down as you age, Facercise can help you counteract this. But, although Facercise will make your face look more toned, it can't restore collagen, the connective fibers in skin that give it elasticity. Unfortunately, nothing can restore collagen as you age.

Here's the briefing that I give all my clients regarding what happens to your face as it ages:

- Skin tone grows paler or yellow
- Nose continues to grow longer and/or wider
- Lips grow thinner
- Eyebrows and eyelids droop
- Under-eye puffiness increases
- Jawline sags and jowls develop
- Mouth corners sag or turn down
- Chin sags; double chin can develop
- Skin on neck grows loose and crepey

If this list makes you feel like begging Ivana Trump for the name of her surgeon or swallowing a bottle of sleeping pills, hold on! The good news is that by doing the exercises in this book, you can expect the following results:

- Rosier skin tone
- Raised or lifted eyebrows
- Enlarged eye sockets, making eyes look more open
- Diminished puffiness under the eyes
- A shorter or narrower nose

- Fuller lips
- Firm jawline, diminished jowls
- Turned-up, young-looking mouth corners
- Toned and smoothed chin and neck

In addition, increased blood circulation and oxygen flow throughout the skin and facial muscles will bring about a rapid improvement in skin color. Sallow, yellow skin, or chalky white complexions will change to fresh, glowing, rosy tones. In my experience, the skin tone transformations are most notable in Asian faces that are yellowish-gray. (My work in Tokyo has been especially exciting because Japanese complexions bloom so quickly.)

Facercise has brought me profound professional and personal fulfill- ment, and it's a pleasure to share my program with you in this book. If you read this book carefully and do the exercises properly, you will see and feel great changes in your face and vitality. Ultimately, Facercise will benefit body and soul. Remember that your mind can make your face more beautiful. Now, that's what I call powerful!

2

WHAT IS FACERCISE?

How and Why It Works

Like me, you've probably looked at people's faces all your life and said to yourself, "That woman is blessed with good bone structure," or "She has great cheekbones, no wonder she's so beautiful." Of course, good bone structure is a key component of facial beauty, but few people realize what an important role facial muscles play in molding the contours of the face. Do you realize that without facial muscles, you could never smile, blink, or frown? Nor could you sneeze, laugh, or yawn.

Muscles in the face are smaller and thinner than most other muscles in the body. But because the fat-to-muscle ratio in the face is lower than it is in most other parts of the body, developed facial muscles can become quite visible from underneath, giving your face a firm and more finely sculpted appearance. I've seen dramatic results achieved in a much shorter time than it takes for changes to appear in, say, the thighs or stomach.

The fact is, facial muscles are terribly under-used: people exercise their bodies, not their faces. Naturally, it follows that most people have weak facial muscles, which invariably sag. And when the muscles sag, the skin attached to them also sags. (You know what an upper arm with an undeveloped tricep looks like?) In fact, slack facial muscles are one of the main causes of the sagging and drooping that most of us eventually experience.

Sagging is a result of the inevitable reduction in collagen and elastin—the skin's connective fibers—as we age. These fibers give skin elasticity and suppleness, and there's no way to restore these substances. Shrinkage of diminished subcutaneous fat, or fat under the skin, also contributes to sagging. Fat reserves under the skin grow smaller with age, and this can partially account for that mid-life "gaunt" look that hollows out an aging face.

Sagging produces bags under the eyes, loose folds of skin on the upper eyelids, pouches, jowls, and turkey necks. Lack of exercise makes the muscle tissue thin and wasted. Working isolated facial muscles with Facercise helps restore muscle tissue's elasticity and tone, making it plump and renewing strength. Like biceps, pectorals, or abdominal muscles, facial muscles must be exercised in order to be firm, fit, and strong.

Muscles are fibrous masses of tissue that are built of protein. Exercising muscles promotes the thickening and strengthening of muscle fibers. To strengthen a muscle, there must first be enough protein in the diet to ensure muscle growth. The goal of exercise is to make the muscle move repeatedly until it tires and the tissue breaks down; after this point rest is essential so that the tissue can regenerate and grow bigger. It's really quite simple: the more a muscle contracts, the more it grows.

With the right balance of exercise and rest, the muscle adapts to the demands placed on it by growing bigger and stronger. Working a muscle to a heightened percentage of its capacity over a relatively short time will increase its size, strength, and ability to contract. By isolating various muscles in the face and performing a repeated range of movements, the muscles are strengthened, regenerated, and enlarged.

You may have heard of—or already tried—other facial exercise programs. Facercise is unique and distinguished by its basic understanding of how muscles work. I've investigated some of these programs; they'll instruct you to do things like open your eyes wide, stick out your tongue, and hold this pose for ten seconds—without any logical explanation of how these various methods work! I can tell you that uninformed programs like these are as useless as those "fat reducing" vibrating machines of the 1950s. Remember those? They had belts that you strapped around your waist so that you could could magically jiggle away unwanted pounds.

No one who is truly interested in building their body would subscribe to this or any other get-fit-quick method. In these health-conscious times, we've become sufficiently aware of what steps need to be taken if one wants to reduce body fat and build muscle: a low-fat diet, an aerobic exercise program, and a careful, applied routine of strength training.

Most of us know that exercises with weights or resistance should be done in multiple sets of eight to twelve repetitions in order to build size and strength. "No pain, no gain," has become an international exercise motto, and, thanks to Jane Fonda, we've all learned to "feel the burn" of working our muscles to the max.

Facercise is the first exercise program to apply these same techniques to the face. When Facercising, you "pump" the muscles around your eyes, for example, the same way you pump iron to develop a more defined chest, a shapelier back, or sculpted arms. Personal trainers talk about the shape, size, and definition of a muscle group; I'm encouraging you to think about the muscles in your face in similar terms.

Isolating and working muscles in the face to the point of feeling a lactic acid burn is the principle behind Facercise. This tingling or burning sensation occurs in a muscle when it is worked to capacity. The muscle produces lactic acid as a result of expending energy and using up ATP, what exercise physiologists and personal trainers call the "energy molecule." Feeling the lactic acid burn tells you that you are making muscles grow stronger and larger.

In the eleven years that I've been teaching, I have consulted with plastic surgeons in order to refine the exercises and make them as effective as possible. Doctors have confirmed my program's safety and integrity, so rest assured that doing Facercise will never overdevelop your facial muscles, a question I'm often asked by skeptics. Believe me, Facercise can only make you look and feel more attractive!

You may also be wondering if Facercise workouts may deepen wrinkles or stretch out your skin. Actually, the *opposite* will occur. As you exercise, you increase blood circulation in the muscles and elsewhere in the face. The result is firmer muscles and taut skin, with smoothed, less visible wrinkles. Although Facercise cannot restore lost collagen or elastin, neither can plastic surgery. (Collagen injections are painful and costly, can leave scars, and must be administered every few months to maintain the puffy look. *Ouch!*) And, unlike plastic surgery, Facercise will greatly improve your skin tone from the inside out.

The program in this book includes fourteen exercises that isolate about thirty of the fifty-seven facial and neck muscles. Because the facial and neck muscles are all interconnected by a network of fibers, however, every muscle benefits.

* * *

Now that I've covered the basic principles of Facercise, I want to explain another reason why Facercise differs from other facial exercise programs. Facercise involves more than performing a workout plan. One of the keys to its effectiveness is that it's the first facial exercise regimen to harness two of your most powerful, renewable assets—your imagination and your energy.

Yes, your mind and your energy play leading roles in making Facercise work. They work together to bring new beauty to your face in what I call the "mind-muscle connection." When I coach my clients, I tell them that they must *feel* their muscles working and *visualize* them growing bigger with every repetition. Devoting your mental and physical powers to these exercises is critically important to your success. You must visualize your muscles growing bigger and stronger with every effort.

Facercise's emphasis on feeling that burning sensation in the muscles is an indication of when you're doing the exercises properly. With such a powerful physical feeling to focus on, your mind stays on track, feeling the muscles grow as you work toward your goals. Your thoughts are as powerful as your actions, and if you *see* and *feel* your muscles enlarging and strengthening as you work, then your face will show the glowing results of your belief and effort.

So remember, when you do your workouts, I want you to be entirely focused on the mind-muscle connection. With these two allies, you can revitalize your face. Facercise provides more than short-term benefits: do your exercises for twenty minutes a day for at least five days a week, and you'll enjoy a lifelong youthful appearance. My hundreds of clients all over the world are living proof of this, and so am I. At forty-nine, I can honestly say that my face is smoother, firmer, rosier, and younger-looking than when I started doing Facercise at age thirty-six. And I've got the photographs to prove it.

The picture on the left was taken when I was thirty-six years old, pre-Facercise. My face was very wrinkled from years of sunbathing; I had wrinkles from the corner of my mouth to the middle of my jaw. I also had a thin, gaunt look because of collagen loss, another result of sun damage. My complexion was gray and not as rosy as I would have liked. My eyebrows were sagging and tired-looking, and my eyes looked small because the upper brows and eyelids were drooping so much. And no amount of makeup could conceal my under-eye bags.

Since I was twenty-one, my face had worn the souvenirs of a bad rhinoplasty. My nose had a hollow on the left side, and the surgeon had also left the nose tip too long, so that it drooped downward. In addition, the surgery had somehow made my upper lip descend and thin out.

Now take a look at the picture on the right—it's me, age forty-nine and it hasn't been retouched! The nasal-labial folds alongside my nose and upper lips have been smoothed out because the muscles underneath my skin are bigger and firmer. The wrinkles are less visible, and my skin tone has changed from gray to a porcelain, pink look. Facercising raised my eyebrows and toned my upper and lower eyelids, making my eyes look larger and more alert.

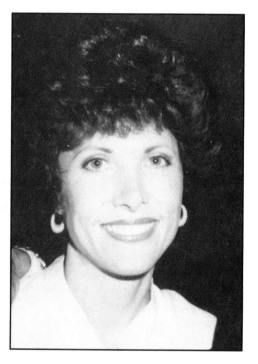

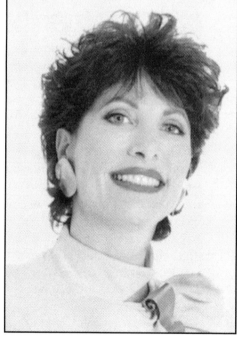

Thanks to my newly developed cheek muscles, my thin face has become fuller and more youthful-looking. My cheeks look firmer and rounder—it felt great to look in the mirror and see a new, sculpted, high-cheekboned face. (I can't tell you how many times people have asked me over the years, "Who did your cheek implants?" When I tell them, "I did," they're confused until I demonstrate by pumping my cheek muscles for them à la Arnold Schwarzenegger!)

To my relief, Facercise made the dent in my nose invisible, and my whole nose looks and feels firmer. I also built up muscle in the nose (yes, folks, there *is* muscle in the nose) so that the tip appears shortened. As for my lips, the upper lip no longer looks so low, and both lips have a fuller, more youthful shape. The corners of my mouth grew stronger and turned up for a younger, smiling, pert look. Another welcome change was a firmer jawline.

I always present these before and after photographs of myself when I go on television to talk about Facercise. Recently I appeared on a television show and a woman who had tuned in called up to tell me, "I saw your photographs and I don't think you look so different." I replied, "Well thank you very much. Those pictures were taken thirteen years apart." The woman signed up for instruction right then and there!

One of the most encouraging sensations of Facercise comes when you actually start to feel the muscles underneath your face. Suddenly you're conscious of that usually dead area between the cheekbones and the mouth, or the space between the ear and nose. Some clients say that after a few days of Facercise, they can feel muscles they didn't know they had. They can feel the exercises are working, and they are encouraged to know that their muscles are growing.

I take a great deal of pride in being able to offer such a healthy, easy, and effective program. And I believe that Facercise owes part of its success to the fact that people have fun doing it. Just imagine, by making faces for a few minutes each day, you can restore youth and vitality to your looks. An easy, enjoyable method for renewing your beauty, the exercises are also effective stress-busters that relax your face, body, and mind.

3

FACIAL AWARENESS

How to Pinpoint and Understand
Your Unique Facial Features

Any discussion of facial characteristics must also consider the nature of most women's self-image—especially *your* self-image. According to a 1994 article in *SELF* magazine, 85 percent of women in the United States admit they don't like their bodies. Now that the global baby boom population is getting older, just imagine how many of them don't like their faces, either! What is your self-image like? How do you honestly feel about your face? Obviously you care about enhancing your appearance, because you're taking the time to read this book. If you're like my clients, you want to look as healthy and youthful as possible. And looking beautiful wouldn't be too bad, either!

But let's get real: very few people possess flawless complexions and beautifully proportioned features. Although heredity is the prime factor that determines your looks, and cosmetic surgery can dramatically alter your features, Facercise is going to help you improve on your assets with an entirely natural method: the mind-muscle connection.

Before you begin your exercises, however, it is critically important that you gain an objective, detailed understanding of your face. You may feel that you know your face very well—better than you'd like to at times! But I want you to be acutely aware of your naturally good features as well as your flaws. Most important, I want you to understand the circumstances that are behind whatever flaws you may have. Then, once we've studied your face in natural light, so to speak, we can start working on enhancing your looks.

I realize that studying your flaws and seeing how your face is aging may make you uncomfortable. But it's the only way to begin. Film stars, models, rock singers, business executives, and royalty have all submitted to this first step. If they can confront their flaws, you can, too! No matter who you are, you owe it to yourself to honestly assess the beauty of your face. This way, instead of hoping for miracles, you can work toward realistic and positive improvements.

The circumstances of your daily life and your living habits directly affect your health and facial appearance. Stop and think about your environment for a moment. Do you live in a dry climate or a damp and cloudy one? Climate can have a detrimental or positive affect on the skin, as can the rhythms of your life. Are you a working mother, always running on a tight schedule? Do you exercise often and take time to relax by yourself? Or are you single and too wrapped up in your career and social life to eat right, sleep regularly, and exercise? If you're stressed out and don't know how to renew your energy, this will show up in your face. Bags under the eyes, under-eye puffiness, pale or gray skin, wrinkles, frown lines and pimples—stress can cause all of these.

God was very smart when he made sure our eyesight gets worse around the same time that our faces begin to drop. It sort of blurs reality, like Vaseline on a lens. But an honest photograph will show exactly what's happened, how you really look, not how you think you look. So the best way to begin is by having someone take a close-up photograph of your face. Take two shots: front and side. Please do *not* smile! These photos will allow you to see your facial contours far more clearly than when you're looking in the mirror. And, they will help you as you work toward correcting your flaws and allow you to observe the progress that you are making as you go along.

These photographs are going to be especially useful to you in the future. Later on, after you have performed your exercises every day for a few weeks, you will take another two photographs from the same distance in the same head-on and side views. Then you can compare before and after and observe the wonderful changes that you have made in your facial features.

Study these photographs of your face very carefully. Every face—even a day-old baby's—has some lines. Without them, a face has no expressive quality. But what kinds of lines do you have? Are they thin or wide? Where are they most concentrated? Also consider how daily living habits can affect your facial appearance. If you've spent years in the sun, as I have, then you probably have fine lines from all that suntanning. If you live on coffee, tea, or soda, and rarely drink water to flush your system, this may account for blemishes, bags under the eyes, or ashen or yellow pallor. Drinking water is one of the best ways to keep skin clear, rosy, and smooth. You'll learn more about how diet affects the skin in Chapter Six, "Your Skin Care Program."

Your emotional tendencies also have a great deal of influence over your facial features. If you worry a lot, this is bound to surface via lines in your forehead and/or around your mouth. Some people question things in their lives so frequently that they form what I call a "question mark line" between the brows. Other people squint habitually, which leads to lines around the eyes.

It's also natural for people to store tension in their faces. Can you see where tension lies in your face? Many of my clients are still quite young, but because they have busy professional and family lives, they constantly look tense and drawn. If you look peaked, Facercise can rapidly help correct this.

Although your personality, energy level, and emotional characteristics influence how your face looks, heredity plays perhaps the biggest role in the formation of facial features and bone structure. It's odd how people's faces can age in the same manner that their parents' did. As I said before, a client will often come to me when her mouth starts looking like her mother's, or when his chin begins to soften like his father's. If you're in either of these camps, relax—doing Facercise can help downplay inherited traits—but you'll have to work at it.

Continue studying the photographs of your face and zero in on your best features and your least attractive ones. What feature do you want to emphasize? Your mouth? Eyes? Cheekbones? Which features do you want to play down? Your nose? Wrinkles? Double chin? Take another long, objective look at your face in the photographs and also determine your face shape. Is it long, round, heart-shaped? If you have full cheeks that are starting to sag in a round face, for instance, you can work at building them up with your Facercise program.

Look at the dramatic results on the following pages achieved after just *six days* of Facercising. Imagine the results after one month.

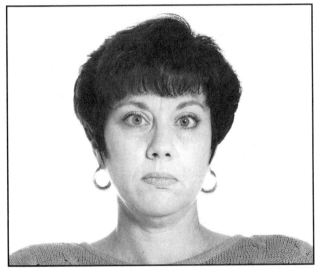

First Day: Sheila has a dull complexion and general lack of muscle tone. Her face shows hollows under her eyes, flat cheeks, a thin upper lip, and sagging mouth corners which make her lower face appear gaunt, along with a heavy nasal labial fold and the beginnings of a double chin.

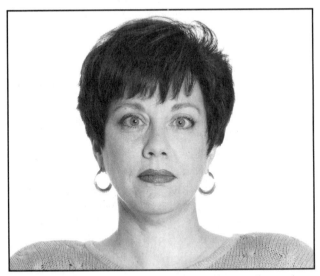

Sixth Day: Her complexion has become more vibrant, the under-eye hollows have faded, the cheeks have grown higher and fuller, the upper lip has filled out, and the mouth corners have turned upward. With a smoother nasal labial fold and a disappearing double chin, her face appears fuller, more defined, and she looks healthier.

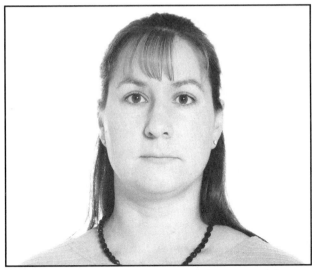

First Day: Dolly's cheeks are flat, she is developing jowls, and the combination of her dull eyes, weak upper lip, and soft jawline give her a look of constant fatigue.

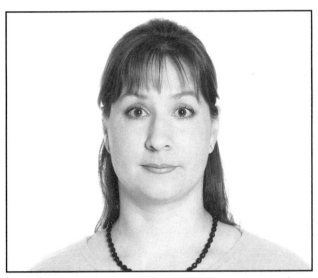

Sixth Day: Her face is more contoured, with higher, fuller cheeks and a tighter jawline. Her upper lip is more defined, and her eyes and overall appearance are more lively.

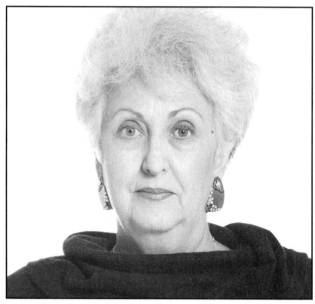

First Day: June's face seems dull, tired, and lacking in overall tone. She suffers from bags under the eyes, low and flat cheeks, a weak upper lip and a fleshy jaw and neckline.

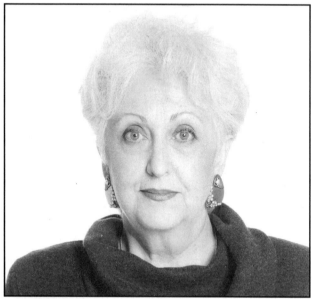

Sixth Day: Diminished under-eye bags, a more defined upper lip, and a tighter jawline and neck make her entire face appear healthier and more toned.

THE TEN MOST–WANTED–GONE LIST

1. *Thin, Hard-Looking Lips*

As you age, the lips and surrounding areas can become very thin and wizened. Tension, smoking, the sun, and habitual facial expressions are the cause of this condition. The resulting lined and sunken effect can add years to your appearance and greatly detract from your beauty. The good news is that this situation can be visibly improved. My exercises will help rebuild the muscles around the mouth, giving a fuller, more youthful look to the face.

2. *Saggy Jawline and/or Double Chin*

Even by the age of thirty or so, your jawline can start to sag, droop, and lose definition, resulting in a weak, vulnerable "grandmother" look. You can greatly improve the tone of your jawline by doing jaw strengthening and neck strengthening exercises. Another benefit you'll reap from doing jawline exercises is renewed confidence—many of my clients find that they speak more authoritatively after they've firmed their face up and reduced their double chin.

3. *Low Eyebrows*

When the muscle tone around the eyes weakens, the area under the eyebrows begins to look droopy and lowered, especially in profile. By doing an exercise that strengthens the eyebrow and scalp muscles so that the brow arch is lifted naturally, you will also strengthen the tiny but vital muscles in the upper eyelids and keep the upper eye area smooth and youthful. Practice the exercises that target this area with dedication and not only your eyes, but your whole face will appear awake and alert.

4. *Drooping Eyelids*

Take it from me—whether you're a drop-dead-gorgeous movie star, a blue-blood queen, or a fresh-scrubbed beauty, there's no escaping it: as you age, your eyelids start to droop. This can also be a hereditary trait—drooping eyelids can run in the family. Besides giving the eyes a hooded appearance, the droops make you look older. With Facercise you will learn a unique method of exercising the eyelids so that their mini-muscles become strong and the eyes open to become larger and more rounded. This creates a more wide-awake, vibrant look, and it will bring sparkle to your eyes. (It's what's earned me the nickname "Starry Eyes"!)

5. Nose Faults

It's very rare that you find someone who's perfectly happy with his or her nose, but let me tell you: large or small, long or short, noses grow larger as people grow older. As cheek muscles slacken and sag, a hollow area is created around the nose. While gravity pulls the nose down, the muscles around the mouth also lose elasticity, which contributes to the sagging. To keep your nose looking young and firm, the most important muscle to build up is the tiny nasal muscle located under each nostril. Exercising this area daily will improve the appearance of the nose as well as the tautness of the mouth and upper lip.

6. Crepey Neck

We've all seen people, even relatively young ones, with creased or crepey-looking throats. This can be caused by too much suntanning, or poor diet combined with lack of exercise. And, of course, plain old aging doesn't help the situation. Because the skin on the throat is delicate, it shows age more easily than other parts of the body. If your neck is thin and the muscles are not in tone, then the problem is compounded. On the brighter side, you can learn how to restore the shape and size of the neck muscles and thus improve the appearance of the entire throat area.

7. Flat Cheeks

Gravity and age work together to flatten out the cheek muscles. As cheek muscles atrophy, the face begins to lose curves and flatten like a tabletop. This casts a tired, older look over the face. The Facercise cheek-enhancing exercises can plump up the muscles so that your cheeks are sculpted and shapely. My clients love these exercises because they invariably help compensate for less-than-perfect bone structure. After you have done these exercises for a few months, the resulting enlarged and strengthened cheek muscles will give your face a firmer, even chiseled look.

* * *

By the time you reach your late twenties, your face is maturing along with your mind and body. All three affect one another and interact to form the personality that one presents to the world. Everyone has three different types of facial lines. By understanding how these lines differ from one another, you will be better able to work on correcting the damage.

8. *Expression Lines*

Emotional reactions to all events and situations in our lives, such as sadness, anger, and even joy, can be recorded in the face as lines—and these lines are not all bad, for they do give us our individual character. All of the Facercise exercises help plump up the underlying muscles of the face, which in turn smooths the skin out and diminishes lines.

9. *Nighttime Furrows*

Sleep lines are what I call the "nighttime enemy." Realize that facial muscles are working even while you sleep—smiling, frowning, and so on. And sleeping with your hands lying under your cheek or burying your face in a scrunched-up pillow will cause cheek furrows. The Facercise cheek exercises will help smooth out the lines that are etched in your face as you sleep.

10. *Wrinkles Due to Loss of Muscle Tone*

The stomach isn't the only part of the body that sags as one grows older. The facial muscles also collapse if they are not properly exercised, and this causes the formation of lines. As we age and lose muscle tone and collagen, the pull of gravity loosens the skin of the face and creates scalloped jowls and lines. Doing regular Facercise will help improve the general tone of all your facial muscles.

CHECKLIST FOR CHANGE

Now that you've considered the pros and cons of your facial features, it's time to get organized. I'd like you to fill in the following checklist. Check the features that you want to improve. Then you will have a program record of what you are going to correct with Facercise. Later, you can compare your exercise results with "before" and "after" photographs.

____ Thin, hard-looking lips/Turned-down mouth corners

____ Saggy jawline/Double chin

____ Low eyebrows

____ Drooping eyelids

____ Long, flabby, or enlarged nose

____ Crepey neck

____ Flat cheeks

____ Expression lines

____ Nighttime furrows

____ Wrinkles due to loss of muscle tone

By now you should have studied your face in close-up and filled out the checklist. Congratulations, you've earned a rest. Take a few minutes to reflect on all the changes that you're going to make in your face, and don't worry if you checked every entry here; you are not alone!

4

THE MUSCLES OF
THE FACE

Where They Are, What They're Called,

How They Work

By now you've committed yourself to making certain changes in your face. With this commitment, you *can* and *will* gain a more youthful-looking appearance. You're almost ready to get started. But first you need to understand where all of your facial muscles are, what they're called, and how these small, interconnected units move. Picture this: beneath your skin, fifty-seven muscles are "wired" together, constantly in motion and at rest. All of these muscles rely upon one another to support and uplift your face.

You may be wondering what this mass of facial muscles looks like. Imagine a magically moving patchwork quilt lying just beneath the surface of your skin. This thin layer of facial muscles is connected by bundles of fibers. I call these muscles magic because of the artistic feats they perform: working with connective fibers, they help express what you feel inside. Without your facial muscles and connective fibers, your face would look like a blank page.

Realize that every time you smile or frown, several muscles team up to

29

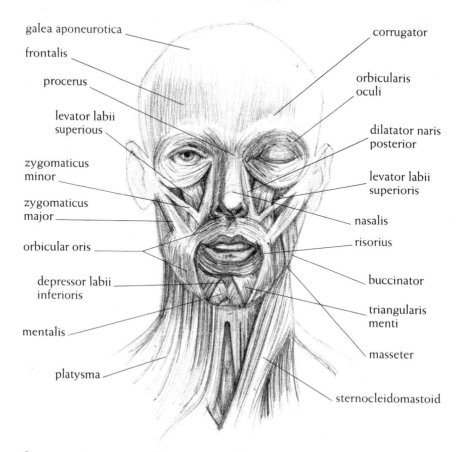

galea aponeurotica

frontalis

procerus

levator labii
superious

zygomaticus
minor

zygomaticus
major

orbicular oris

depressor labii
inferioris

mentalis

platysma

corrugator

orbicularis
oculi

dilatator naris
posterior

levator labii
superioris

nasalis

risorius

buccinator

triangularis
menti

masseter

sternocleidomastoid

form your expression. For instance, the mouth and cheek muscles work with muscles around your eyes and temples when you smile. When you get tense, your scalp muscles work in tandem with muscles in the eyes, and so on and so forth.

When you learn Facercise, it is vital that you practice the exercises as they are numbered, lesson by lesson. To gain optimum results, you must do the exercises in the sequence that they are presented. Why? Because while you're working one set of muscles, you want others to be resting and rebuilding.

Knowing where the various muscles are in the face, visualizing their range of motion and what their jobs are, will help you make that crucial mind-muscle connection. If you can get into this state of mind/body, then you're sure to see good results in your face.

Facercise targets about thirty muscles in the face, neck, and scalp. When developing my program, I isolated these muscles because they decisively influence facial expression and beauty. I want to stress, however, that all fifty-seven facial and neck muscles are interconnected, so they all benefit from Facercise.

The ability to visualize and feel different muscles moving and growing as you work will help you do the exercises with perfect form. And, as you work out, your muscles become so accustomed to their special movements that the exercises gradually become more effective. Take a few minutes to study the following description of your muscles and locate them on the illustration on page 30. Knowing where your muscles are and what they do will help you bring your best face forward.

MUSCLES OF THE SCALP

You may be interested to know that the skin on the scalp is the thickest skin on the body. Underneath this skin, scalp muscles are divided into three areas:

The *frontalis* is a thin muscle located over the forehead. It draws the scalp forward, producing horizontal wrinkles in the forehead.

The *occipitalis* is about an inch and a half long and lies at the back of the head. It pulls the scalp backward.

The *galea aponeurotica* is a broad, flat tendon joining the frontalis and occipitalis muscles.

MUSCLES OF THE MOUTH

The *orbicular oris* completely encircles the mouth. It consists of numerous strands of muscle fibers, which go in different directions and connect with fibers in the upper and lower lips, cheeks, nose, and the surrounding areas.

The *buccinator* is a broad, thin muscle beneath the cheek. It works to compress the cheek, as when you forcefully exhale or whistle.

The *quadratus labii superioris* is a relatively large muscle that lies beneath the upper lip and connects to muscles in the cheek.

The *mentalis* is a tiny muscle in the front of the chin.

The *quadratus menti* is a small four-sided muscle. It draws down the lower lip. Containing much fat intermingled with its fibers, this muscle benefits from exercise by making the lower lip look fuller.

The *triangularis menti* is a triangular-shaped muscle rising from the lower jaw up to the mouth. It helps draw down the corners of the mouth.

The *risorius* is a narrow bundle of muscle fibers that retracts the corners of the mouth toward the back teeth.

The *zygomaticus major* and the *zygomaticus minor* are two muscles comprised of slender cords of muscle fibers that raise the corners of the mouth and extend into the cheek. They are also known as the "laughing muscles" for the role they play when you smile or laugh.

The fibers of the thin *levator labii superioris* muscle converge in the upper lip.

MUSCLES OF THE NOSE

The *pyrimadalis nasi* spans the bridge of the nose. It draws down the middle of the eyebrows and wrinkles the nose.

The *dilatator naris posterior* is a small muscle situated above and behind the nostril. Working this muscle can help re-contour your nose.

The thin and delicate *dilatator naris anterior* lies directly above the middle of each of your nostrils. This is the muscle that causes your nostrils to flare.

The *depressor alae nasi* extends across the base of the nose and closes the nasal opening by pulling down the septum.

The *compressor nasi* begins at the bridge of the nose and extends up over the bridge, compressing the nostrils.

MUSCLES OF MASTICATION

Mastication is the opening and closing of the jaws, such as when chewing and yawning. Many people hold tension in their jaws, and knowing where these muscles are and how to work them can help you relax, as well as build up muscle tone in the face.

The *temporal* is a large muscle on the side of the head that closes the jaws with force. It goes diagonally back from the cheekbone to the outer jaw hinge.

A short, thick muscle, the *masseter* works in conjunction with the *temporal* to clench the jaws. Working this muscle helps firm up slack jawlines and double chins.

Short, thick, and cone-shaped, the *external pterygoid* helps to close the mouth and rotate the jaw.

The *pterygoid internus* also helps to close the mouth and move the jaw. Exercising this muscle will help create a well-toned jawline.

What I refer to as the "double chin" muscle, the *digastricus* runs from the chin into the top of the neck.

MUSCLES OF THE EYE

The *levator palpebra superioris* in the upper eyelid is extremely thin but vital to maintaining firm, toned upper eyelids.

The *orbicularis oculi* is a powerful muscle that surrounds the orbit of the eye. You couldn't see much without it, as it acts to open and close the eye. And you couldn't look surprised without it, because it helps raise your eyebrows! When you squint, the *orbicularis oculi* raises the lower eyelid.

The *corrugator* muscle juts out from the top of the forehead and runs into the muscle within the upper eyelid. Building this one can help smooth out forehead lines.

The *epicranius* raises the eyebrows. Working this muscle helps increase oxygen and blood circulation throughout the forehead and eyes. Regular exercise of the epicranius can also soften tense brows, making you look more relaxed.

MUSCLES OF THE NECK

The *platysma* is a broad, thin plane of muscular fibers lying beneath the skin on each side of the neck. A powerful muscle, it works to depress the lower jaw.

The *sterno-cleido-mastoid* rotates the head and draws it to either side.

The *trapezius* lies at the back of the head and shoulders and draws the head back and from side to side.

MUSCLES OF THE EAR

The following three muscles lie immediately underneath the skin around the ear. Although they have relatively little influence on facial appearance, these muscles are connected to the muscles that you work while Facercising. Most important, learning how to make these muscles move will help strengthen and define your scalp and face muscles. When you're doing exercises that firm your jawline, for instance, think about flexing the ears—this will help you work the jaw muscle group. Also, when you're doing exercises that lift and tone the upper eye and eyebrow area, flexing the ears will help lessen frown lines around the eyes.

The *anterior auricular* is the smallest ear muscle. Thin and fan-shaped, it draws the ears forward.

The largest ear muscle, the *superior auricular,* raises the ears.

The *posterior auricular* draws the ear backward.

Now that you know the names and locations of various muscles, you're ready to start working them via Facercise. You now possess both the vehicle and the map that will help you attain a more beautiful appearance. After learning the exercises in the following chapter, you can hit the road.

5

THE EXERCISES

HOW TO SUCCEED AT FACERCISE

The Facercise program teaches you new skills that are gradually perfected through daily practice. Once you've memorized the fourteen exercise movements, doing them becomes second nature. After a few months of daily workouts, you will be experienced enough to start doing advanced versions of the exercises.

The great advantage of Facercise is that it's a flexible program that you can do anywhere or anytime. At the end of this chapter is a section that explains how to do a modified version of Facercise when you're driving. I Facercise throughout the course of each day—when I'm talking on the phone, studying a menu in a restaurant, doing housework, or watching television. As you learn the exercises in this chapter, you'll find out how easy it is to work Facercise into your day, no matter where you may be.

As with all health and fitness programs, it is essential that you schedule Facercise into your daily life and establish the right routine from the very start. I suggest doing the exercises in the morning for eleven minutes and at night for eleven minutes. To obtain the best results, you must do each of the exercises every day, twice a day, while you are learning them—

and for six to eight weeks thereafter. Remember, good Facercise habits will help you re-contour and tone your face quickly.

Most of my clients find that after a few months of disciplined work-outs, they've knocked anywhere from five to ten years off their appearance. And believe me, people will begin to notice. There are no shortcuts in Facercise, but as I've said before, the exercises are fun and totally portable. And once you achieve the changes that you were seeking, you may advance to a "maintenance" program. This means doing your exercises every other day—or as your face needs them.

Got all that? Good. Store it in your memory bank. Now I want to wish you the best of luck with Facercise, and give you a gentle reminder. Get familiar with Facercise methods by reading through all of the exercise directions two or three times before committing to the program. As you read, visualize and practice doing the exercises. You'll soon be on your way to a more radiant, youthful face.

A NOTE ON MY EXERCISE METHOD

One of the basic premises of Facercise is that you focus on the muscle as you work it to the point where you feel a lactic acid burn. The fingers or fingertips are often placed on top of the muscles of the face to function as counterweights: the weight of the fingers provides resistance and helps maintain focus. This makes the muscles work harder and grow bigger and stronger as quickly as possible.

Another exercise tip is to feel and visualize the energy that flows through your muscles as you work. When you read the exercise instructions that follow, you will see that I often say things like "Follow the energy in your face." My concept of energy flow is based on traditional Chinese medicine's theory that energy moves in pathways throughout the body. I also believe that there is an energy field around your body. I know from experience that feeling and visualizing energy flows and energy fields helps people learn and memorize the exercises more quickly. The big payoff is that visualizing energy leads to more rapid muscle development than you get when you exercise without your imagination.

When I mention energy and energy flows in the exercise instructions, I also often tell the exerciser to "pulse" with the fingers or make "pulsing" motions. By "pulse," I mean make a rapid up-and-down movement. Pulsing helps you feel and see energy, intensify the burn, and perform the exercises with maximum concentration and correct form.

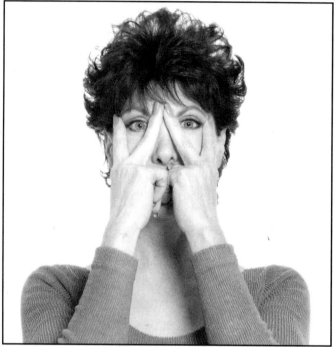

FIGURE 1

Exercise #1
EYE ENHANCER

RESULTS: The Eye Enhancer exercises the *orbicularis oculi* muscle that surrounds the entire eye. One of the most important muscles in the body, the
orbicularis oculi opens and closes the eyes. This exercise pumps blood into
the whole eye area and strengthens the upper and lower eyelids. It also
reduces under-eye puffiness, lifts under-eye hollows, and in effect enlarges
the eye socket, giving you a more wide-awake, bright-eyed look. You may
be wondering how the eye socket can be enlarged. Here are the facts: as
you age, the upper eyelid muscle loses tone and sags down on the eye
socket, invading the area and making it smaller. When you tone and lift the
upper and lower eyelids, the eye socket is enlarged and made more defined.

METHOD: Do this exercise lying down or in a sitting position. Place your
middle fingers between the brows, above the bridge of your nose. Place
your index fingers at your outer eye corners (fig. 1). Make a strong squint *up*
with the lower eyelid—feel the outer eye muscle pulse. Squint and release

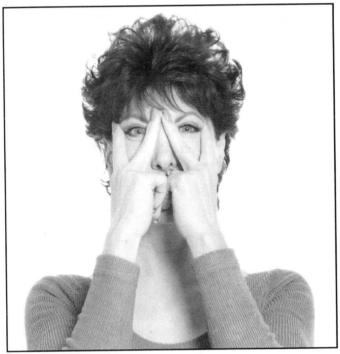

FIGURE 2

ten times, focusing on the pulsing each time you squint (fig. 2). Now hold the squint and squeeze your eyes tightly shut while counting up to forty. Focus your mind on the outer eye muscle pulsing. Be sure to keep eyes squeezed shut very tight as you count.

REMEMBER: Do the Eye Enhancer exercise twice a day. Try it three times a day to correct deep hollows or severe under-eye puffiness, under-eye droop, or to enlarge the eye socket.

MEMO: In the morning, if your eyes are puffy and you haven't had time to Facercise, do two Eye Enhancers and then apply your makeup. This will brighten your eyes considerably and remove the look of fatigue.

ADVANCED METHOD: After you have mastered the above exercise, try this one, which will bring you greater results faster. Do this exercise lying down. Each time you squint and release, lift your head off the bed or floor a half inch to make the muscle work harder. On the tenth squint, hold the squint and squeeze your eyes shut tight and count to twenty. Then raise your head a half inch, continuing to keep your eyes shut tight, and count another twenty.

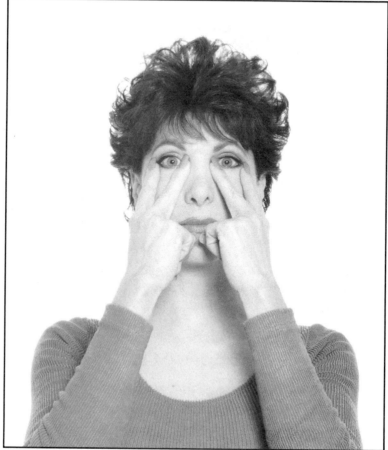

FIGURE 1

Exercise #2
LOWER EYELID STRENGTHENER
∽⊗∾

RESULTS: This exercise also strengthens the *orbicularis oculi*, firming the lower eyelid, diminishing the hollows under the eyes, and reducing under-eye puffiness.

METHOD: This exercise may be done sitting or lying down. Place an index finger at the outer corner of each eye, and your middle fingers at the inner eye corners (fig. 1). Squint strongly with your lower eyelids, thinking *up*. Feel your outer and inner eye muscles flex (fig. 2). Squint and release ten

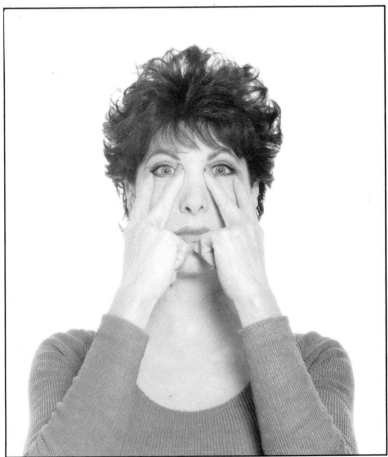

FIGURE 2

times, keeping your upper eyelids open wide. Now hold the squint and think *up*, maintaining the strong squint with your lower eyelids as you count to forty, focusing on the outer and inner eye muscles flexing. Repeat the entire exercise.

REMEMBER: Perform the Lower Eyelid Strengthener twice a day. If you have excessive under-eye puffiness, repeat three times a day.

ADVANCED METHOD: Do this exercise lying down. Each time you squint and release, raise your head a half inch off the bed or floor. Hold squint count for twenty, then raise your head a half inch off the floor again and count another twenty.

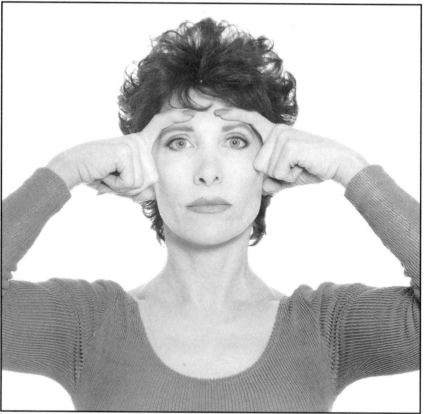

FIGURE 1

Exercise #3
FOREHEAD LIFT

RESULTS: This multipurpose exercise works the *epicranius*, which raises the eyebrows, the *frontalis*, which draws the scalp forward, the *occipitalis*, which draws the scalp back, and the *galea aponeurotica*, which joins the *frontalis* and the *occipitalis*. The Forehead Lift mercifully prevents, or reduces, the frown lines between the eyebrows, and also raises the eyebrows. As well, it prevents or diminishes hooding of the upper eyelids.

METHOD: Try this in a sitting position or lying down. Place the index fingers of both hands high on the forehead so that one of them is parallel to the top of each brow (fig. 1). Now pull the fingers down so that they're approximately a half inch above the brows. While fingers are pressing

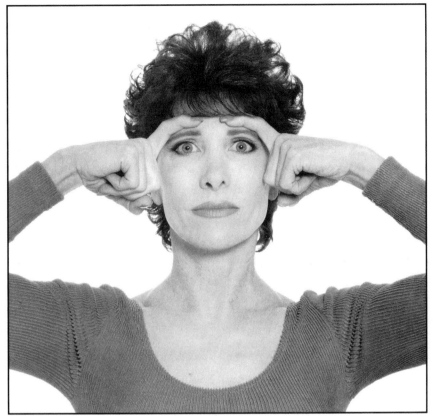

FIGURE 2

down, concentrate on pushing the eyebrows up (fig. 2). Push eyebrows up and release ten times. Now hold eyebrows in up position, continuing to keep fingers pressed down—and do mini-eyebrow push-ups until you feel a tight band of pressure above the brows. Hold them up and count to twenty. Release.

REMEMBER: Do the Forehead Lift twice a day. It helps to clear the head and make you feel more alert. To correct a heavy or scowling brow, do it three times a day.

ADVANCED METHOD: Do the exercise lying down. Raise your head off the bed or floor a half inch each time you push up eyebrows and release. Feel the band of pressure across your forehead. On the final push-up, raise head a half inch and count to twenty.

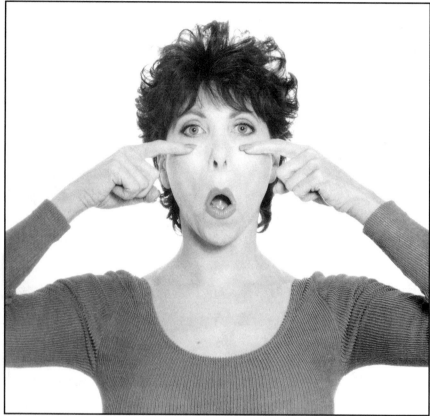

FIGURE 1

Exercise #4

CHEEK DEVELOPER

RESULTS: The Cheek Developer exercises the *buccinator* muscle. This is the rounded top part, or "apple," of the cheek. The exercise also works the *orbicular oris*, which is the circular muscle surrounding the mouth. It lifts and enlarges the cheeks and removes hollows from under the eyes.

METHOD: Do this exercise in either a sitting position or lying down. Place an index finger on top of the apple of each cheek. Open your mouth and pull the upper and lower lips away from each other, forming a long, strong O shape. Hold the long O shape of the mouth firmly in place. Keep the upper lip pressing down against the teeth (fig. 1). Smile with your mouth

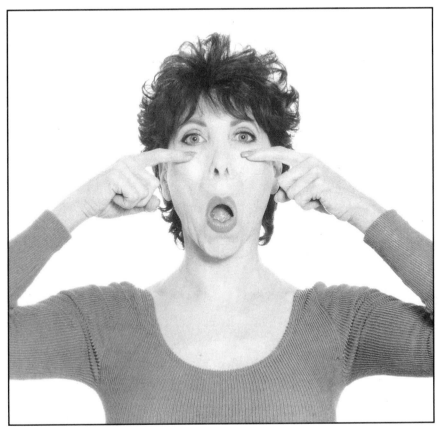

FIGURE 2

corners and release (fig. 2). Repeat thirty-five times, feeling the cheek muscles move under your index fingers. Use your mind-muscle connection and *visualize* that you're pushing the muscles up under the cheeks each time you smile. Your cheek muscles will really feel like they're working as you exercise. And after doing the Cheek Developer, your face will feel energized.

REMEMBER: Perform the Cheek Developer at least two times daily. You can easily do this exercise while walking around the house or watching television.

ADVANCED METHOD: You guessed it—this is another head raiser. Lift your head off the floor a half inch each time you smile and flex your cheeks.

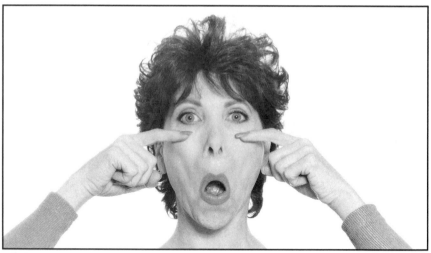

FIGURE 1

Exercise #5
FACE ENERGIZER

RESULTS: I want you to know that although the Face Energizer may sound similar to the Cheek Developer, there is one crucial difference. Yes, the Cheek Developer makes cheeks fuller. But the Face Energizer uses the mind-muscle connection to combat the lengthening and flattening effects of gravity. The exercise encourages the muscles in the cheeks and mouth to work against gravity's downward pull. It also helps remove the hard look of stress from the face and greatly increases blood circulation, giving your complexion a rosy glow.

METHOD: While lying down, pull the upper and lower lips apart, opening the mouth to form a long O. Place index fingers on top of cheeks for light resistance, and keep your upper lip pressed down against the teeth (fig. 1). Smile with your mouth corners and release ten times, feeling the cheeks move under the index fingers. Visualize pushing the muscle up under the cheek each time you smile. On the tenth smile, use all your strength to pull the upper and lower lips away from each other. Imagine your cheeks are moving *out* from your face and *up* toward the ceiling, *out through the top of your scalp*. Hold for a count of thirty. Take index fingers a half inch away from the face, then start to move fingers up in front of the face, toward the scalp (fig. 2). (This helps you move the energy field around the body as you *visualize* cheeks moving up through the top of the head.) Now, raise

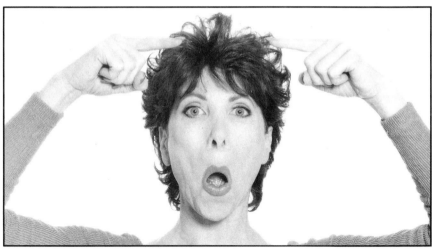

FIGURE 2

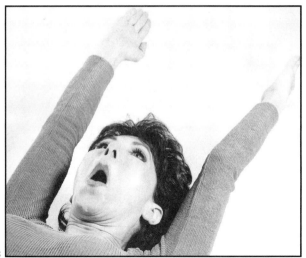

FIGURE 3

your head one inch, hold it up, and count to thirty, continuing to imagine that your cheeks are moving up and out of the top of your head (fig. 3).

REMEMBER: Do your Face Energizer two times a day. If you're under stress, do it more often. Some people feel an ache in their faces the day after they've done this exercise for the first two times. This is a sign that the muscle is getting stronger.

ADVANCED METHOD: Do a head raiser a half inch off the bed or floor as you smile and release ten times, flexing the cheek muscles all the while. Continue the exercise as described above.

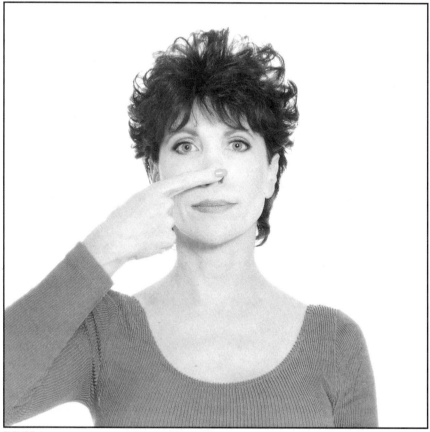

FIGURE 1

Exercise #6
NOSE SHORTENER

RESULTS: As I've said before, the nose is fated to grow throughout our lives, and the tip drops and widens with age. The good news is that the Nose Shortener shortens and narrows the nose tip by exercising the *dilator naris posterior* and *dilator naris anterior*. This is how I fixed my fixed nose.

METHOD: In a sitting position or lying down, use the forefinger to push the tip of the nose up and hold firmly in place (fig. 1). Flex your nose down by pulling your upper lip down over the teeth, holding for a second before releasing the lip (fig. 2). Repeat thirty-five times, feeling the nose tip push against the finger each time. Remember to keep breathing at a steady rate

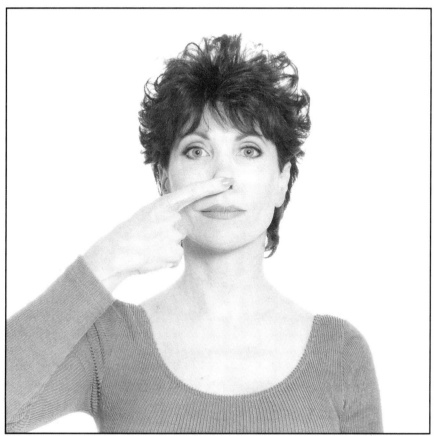

FIGURE 2

while you do the repetitions. This will aid your concentration as you work. Doing this exercise properly stimulates blood and oxygen flow in your upper lip and nose. Many of my clients describe feeling a tingling around the nose, which is a result of increased blood circulation. You'll feel relaxed and clearheaded after doing thirty-five reps of the Nose Shortener.

MEMO: Some of my clients who have had rhinoplasty surgery report that doing this exercise for several weeks helps give their nose a more naturally sculpted look.

REMEMBER: Do the Nose Shortener once a day, twice if you're shortening a very long nose or narrowing a wide nose.

ADVANCED METHOD: Lying down, do a head raiser a half inch off the bed or floor each time while pulling down the upper lip and releasing it.

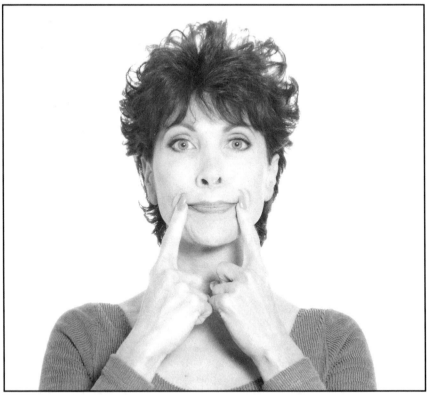

FIGURE 1

Exercise #7
MOUTH CORNER LIFT

RESULTS: With age, the *zygomaticus* muscles sag, causing the mouth corners to droop. This exercise causes droopy mouth corners to firm up and turn up.

METHOD: This exercise can be done sitting or lying down. Close your lips together. Tighten the corners of your mouth into hard knots by sucking them in tight to the back teeth. Never clench your teeth, and maintain steady breathing as you go. Place your index fingers lightly on the corners of your mouth (fig. 1). Keep sucking the corners of your mouth in and *visualize* the corners turning up in a tiny smile, then *visualize* the corners turning down like a tiny frown. *Imagine* turning them slowly up and down. Continue visualizing the corners going up and down. Move your fingers

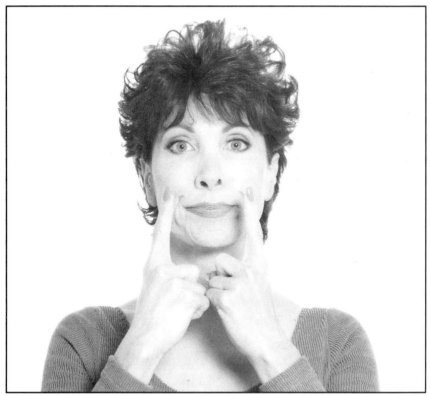

FIGURE 2

away from the corners of your mouth in tiny up-and-down pulses, following the energy you feel in the corners (fig. 2). Continue moving the fingers away until the muscles at the corners of the mouth burn. Hold the burn for a count of twenty, moving the fingers up and down in half-inch pulses. Believe me, this will intensify the burn.

REMEMBER: The success of this exercise relies heavily on your use of the mind-muscle connection. In your mind, you are visualizing the corners of your mouth going up and down about a half inch as you pulse the index fingers. This is a mental movement, not a physical movement! Do the Mouth Corner Lift exercises twice daily.

ADVANCED METHOD: Do a head raiser a half inch off the bed each time you visualize the corners moving up and down. When you feel the burn, keep your head up and count to thirty, pulsing the fingers up and down.

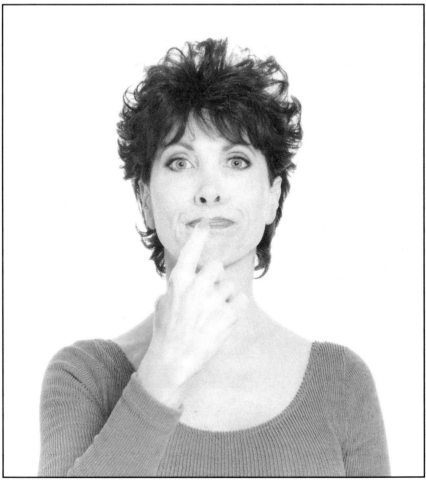

FIGURE 1

Exercise #8
LIP SHAPER

RESULTS: By working the *orbicular oris* muscle around the mouth, the Lip Shaper makes the mouth look younger, firmer, and fuller. This exercise enlarges the lips and smoothes out lines above the upper lip.

METHOD: This can be done sitting up or lying down. Close your lips. Don't clench your teeth. Put the tip of your index finger in between your upper and lower lips. Press lips together and visualize your finger as a

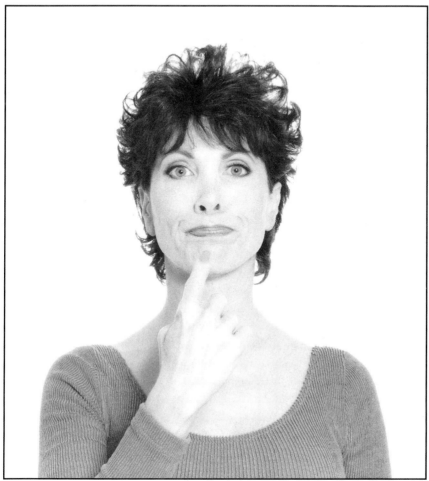

FIGURE 2

pencil that you are crushing (fig. 1). Slowly pull your finger out from the center of your lips while seeing and feeling the pencil. Draw the energy point out and lengthen your imaginary pencil until you feel the burn (fig. 2). Pulse your finger up and down quickly for a count of thirty.

REMEMBER: Do the Lip Shaper twice a day to plump up thin lips. This is a healing exercise for people who hold their tension in their mouths.

ADVANCED: Do this lying down and raise your head one inch off the bed or floor as soon as you feel the burn. Hold and pulse the finger quickly up and down to intensify the burn for a count of thirty.

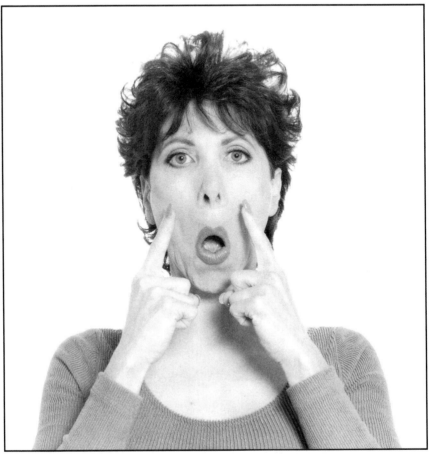

FIGURE 1

Exercise #9
NASAL LABIAL SMOOTHER

RESULTS: This little workout can help make a big improvement in your appearance. By building up the *dilator anterior* and the *dilator posterior* muscles, you will plump up deep creases and smooth out age lines from the nose to the corners of the mouth.

METHOD: This works best when sitting in an upright position. Pull your upper and lower lips away from each other to open your mouth into a long O (fig. 1). Pull your upper mouth corners up into a smile—use only your upper lip. Wrinkle your nose *upward* like a rabbit while smiling with

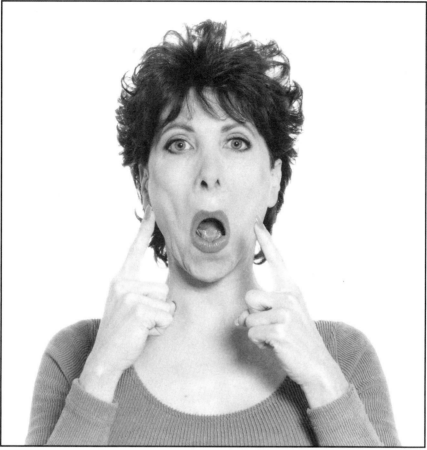

FIGURE 2

the upper lip. Keeping your upper lip pressed against your teeth, push the upper lip down hard (fig. 2). You will feel the pull along the sides of the nose. It's important that you wrinkle the nose up rabbit-style with each smile or curl of the upper lip—this forces energy to keep moving along the sides of the nose. Use your fingertips to trace and intensify the lines of energy along the sides of the nose up and down. Keep moving the energy up and down until you feel the burning sensation along the nasal labial fold. Hold the position, keeping your nose wrinkled, and quickly pulse the fingers up and down for a count of twenty.

REMEMBER: Using your mind-muscle connection on this one helps intensify the burn and develop the muscle more quickly. Do the Nasal Labial Smoother twice a day, or more if your facial lines are deeply etched.

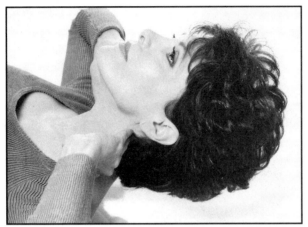

FIGURE 1

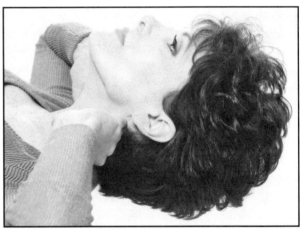

FIGURE 2

Exercise #10
NECK STRENGTHENER

RESULTS: This exercise strengthens the *platysma, sterno-cleido-mastoid,* and the *trapezius*—all the muscles of the neck. Besides helping to strengthen these important muscles that keep our heads upright, working them will firm up and smooth out the skin, counteracting sagging neck skin. After a few days of doing the Neck Strengthener, your neck will feel stronger, allowing you to hold your head higher. And this can help your posture—as well as your confidence.

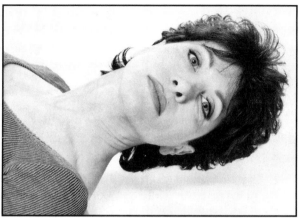

FIGURE 3

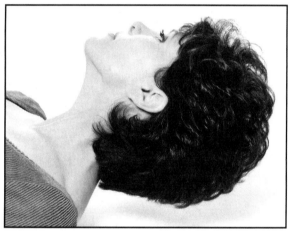

FIGURE 4

METHOD: This exercise works best lying down. Grasp the sides of your neck under the ears with your fingertips. Press your fingertips into the neck (fig. 1). Raise your head a half inch off the bed, leading with the front of your neck, then lower (fig. 2). Repeat twenty-five times, feeling how your neck muscles flex each time. Place your hands down at the sides of your body, lift your head and shoulders off the bed, turn your head side to side, then lower back to the bed each time before doing another repetition (figs. 3 & 4). Repeat twenty times.

REMEMBER: Do the Neck Strengthener once a day if your neck is thick, and twice a day if it is long and thin.

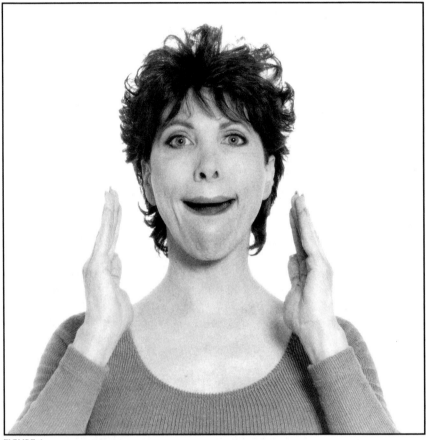

FIGURE 1

Exercise #11
JAW STRENGTHENER

RESULTS: This exercise benefits the *pterygoid internus* muscle in the jaw. Working this muscle pulls up droopy jowls and erases sagging, scallopy skin around the jawline.

METHOD: In a sitting position, open your mouth and roll your lower lip in tight over the lower teeth. Pull the corners of your mouth to the back and keep them rolled in tightly. Keep your upper lip pressed against your teeth (fig. 1). Open and close your jaw in a slow, scooping motion using the *corners* of your mouth to open and close the lower jaw, imagining picking

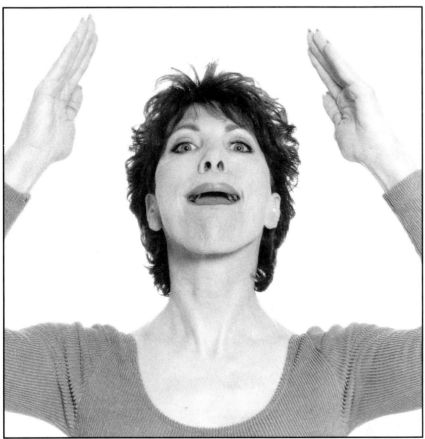

FIGURE 2

something up with your jaw as you scoop. Pull your chin up a half inch as you scoop. *Visualize* the sides of the face lifting up. Place your hands a half inch away from the sides of your face to help move up the energy field of the face. At this point, your head will be tilted back and your chin should be pointing toward the ceiling (fig. 2). Scoop slowly and concentrate on *visualizing* the sides of your face lifting. After doing about six deliberate scoops, you should feel a burn. When you feel the burn, hold the pose and count to twenty.

REMEMBER: Do your Jaw Strengthener at least two times a day. Along with improving your appearance, it will also work to arrest further sagging.

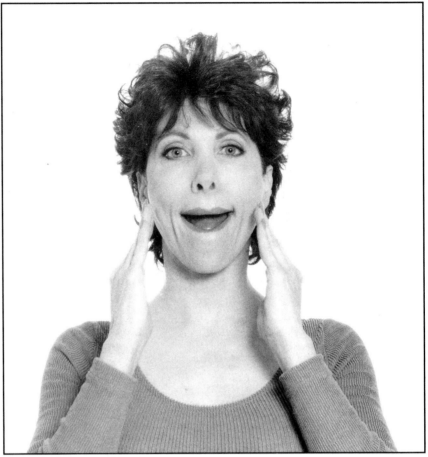

FIGURE 1

Exercise #12
FACE WIDENER

RESULTS: Especially helpful for long, narrow faces, this works several muscles and helps fill out sunken cheeks. It helps widen the face and softens the thin, gaunt, "witchy" look.

METHOD: You can do this sitting up or lying down. First, open your mouth and pull the mouth corners to the back teeth and roll them in like tight anchors. Keep your upper lip pressed down against the upper teeth (fig. 1). *Visualize* big, fat cheeks coming out of the corners of your mouth and filling

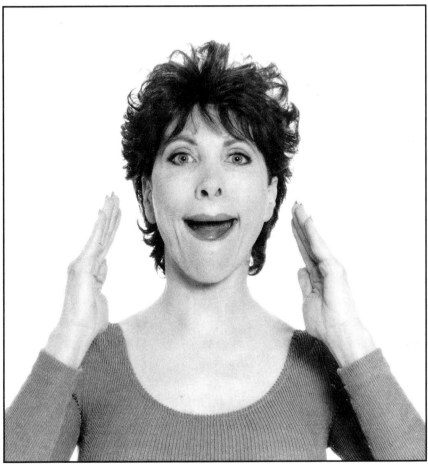

FIGURE 2

in the gaunt area. Place your fingertips on your mouth corners and slowly pull fingers away from the sides of your face. Keep the corners of your mouth rolled in and pulled back (fig. 2). Continue slowly pulling the fingers away until you feel the muscles burn, then raise your head about one inch. Hold it there and count to thirty-five. At this point, keep your hands about two inches away from the sides of your face and make quick small circles with the hands to intensify the burn.

REMEMBER: The Face Widener should be done twice a day to correct a narrow or gaunt face. Skip this exercise if you think that your face is too wide.

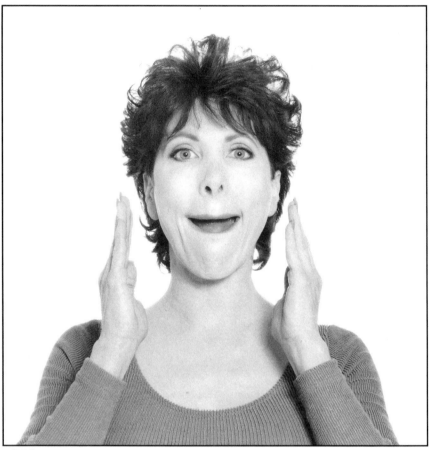

FIGURE 1

Exercise #13
FACE SLIMMER

RESULTS: The Slimmer narrows, lifts, and tones a wide face. Exercising the *buccinator* muscle will increase facial muscle tone. If your face is thin, do this exercise only once a day.

METHOD: Try this sitting up or lying down. Open your mouth and force-fully roll your lips over your teeth. Pull the corners of your mouth to the back teeth and roll them in tightly (fig. 1). Use your mind-muscle connection and *visualize* the sides of your face moving up and out past the jawline

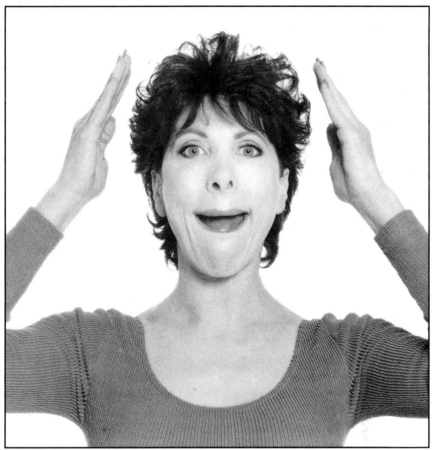

FIGURE 2

to the top of the head. Place one hand on each side of your face and slowly move hands up along the sides of your face as you visualize your face lifting (fig. 2). Continue until you feel the burn. Hold and, if you're lying down, raise head one inch, count to thirty.

REMEMBER: Do the Face Slimmer twice a day for a heavy, full face or for heavy sagging.

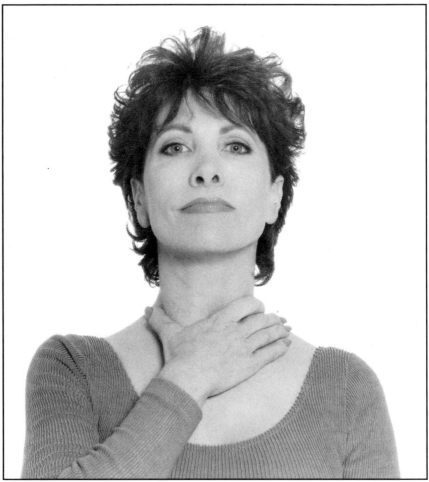

FIGURE 1

Exercise #14
NECK AND CHIN TONER

RESULTS: Great for firming the chin, neck, and jawline, this exercise works and strengthens the *platysma* muscle. It can greatly reduce double chins, and in some cases, can make them almost invisible.

METHOD: Sit tall and straight with your chin held high. Close your lips and smile *only* with your upper lip. Place one hand at the base of the throat,

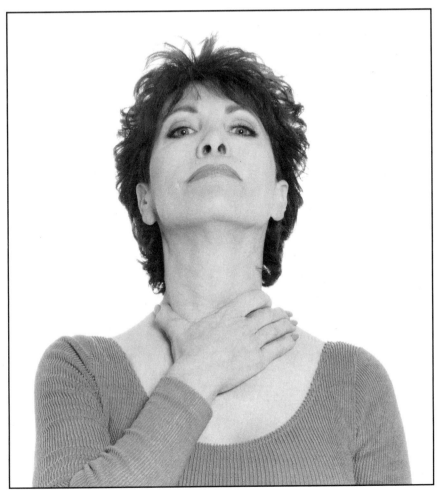

FIGURE 2

over the collarbone, and pull down slightly on the skin with a firm grip (fig. 1). Tilt your head back to feel a strong pull on the chin and neck muscles (fig. 2), then release. Repeat thirty times.

REMEMBER: Do the Neck and Chin Toner more often than twice daily if it is a problem area.

KEEP FACERCISING

Because I want you to reach your goals, I want to stress again that Facercise is a versatile improvement program. You can fit in your exercises anytime, anywhere. These days, everyone's spare time is precious. Whenever you've got free time is the right time to Facercise. I've adapted the following exercises so that they can be done easily—and safely—while driving.

DOING FACERCISE IN THE CAR

My clients who drive say that they get quite a boost from doing Facercise behind the wheel. Along with making Facercisers look and feel more youthful, the exercises help clear the head and improve concentration. Doing Facercise in your car may bring you other bonuses, as the following anecdote illustrates.

I had a client in her mid-fifties who Facercised religiously in her car. One day she was doing the exercises at a stoplight. When she arrived at her destination, a handsome man in his thirties pulled up alongside her as she got out of her car. "Excuse me," he said, "I was driving behind you and saw you smiling at me in the rearview mirror at the stoplight."

The woman laughed and explained that she had been doing facial exercises. The man was intrigued, and when she told him her age, he couldn't believe it. He asked her to tell him more, and at the end of their conversation, they'd made a date. Despite their difference in ages, those two were a couple for quite some time after that. If only Facercising in the car could net every woman a handsome younger man! But seriously, the point of this story is to forget your self-consciousness and do your exercises in the car. They will make the most of your free time and can yield unanticipated benefits.

CAR EXERCISE #1: EYE ENHANCER

Do this while waiting at a stoplight or when you're stopped in bumper-to-bumper traffic. Place your middle fingers between the brows. Place your index fingers at your outer eye corners. Forcefully squint up with the lower eyelid—feel the outer eye muscle pulse. Squint and release ten times. Focus on the pulsing each time you squint. Now hold the squint, and squeeze your eyes shut while counting to forty. Peek with one eye every few counts to check if the light has changed, and continue squeezing!

CAR EXERCISE #2: LOWER EYELID STRENGTHENER

You can do this while driving or stopped in traffic. Place your left thumb at the outer corner of the left eye and your left index finger at the outer corner of the right eye. Squint up and release ten times, feeling the outer eye muscles pulse. Hold for a count of forty, keeping upper eyelid open wide while pushing away from the steering wheel with your other hand. Then place your thumb and index finger at the inner eye corners. Squint up and release ten times. Then hold for a count of forty, still pushing against the steering wheel.

CAR EXERCISE #3: FOREHEAD LIFT

The Forehead Lift can be done while driving or stopped in traffic. Place the thumb and index finger of one hand on top of each brow and pull your fingers down so that they're pushing down against the brows. Push your eyebrows up and release ten times. Now hold your eyebrows up, keeping the fingers pulled down, until you feel the band of pressure across your forehead. Hold and count to twenty.

CAR EXERCISE #4: CHEEK DEVELOPER

Place the thumb and index finger of one hand on top of one cheek. Open your mouth and pull the upper and lower lips away from each other, forming a long, strong O shape. Keep the long O shape of the mouth strong. Keep the upper lip pressing down against the teeth. Smile with your mouth corners and release. Repeat thirty-five times, feeling the cheek muscle move under your thumb and finger. Use your mind-muscle connection and visualize that you're pushing the muscle up under the cheek each time you smile. Repeat exercise on the other cheek. You'll feel your cheek muscles pumping as you exercise, and as blood circulation increases while you work, your cheeks will feel energized.

CAR EXERCISE #5: FACE ENERGIZER

While driving, pull the upper and lower lips apart, opening the mouth to form a long O. Use the thumb and index finger of one hand on top of the cheeks. Smile with your mouth corners and release ten times, feeling the cheeks move under the thumb and index finger. Imagine that you're pushing the muscle up under the cheek each time you smile. On the tenth smile, forcefully pull the upper and lower lip away from each other. Visualize that you're pushing your cheeks out toward the windshield, then up and out of the roof of the car. Count to forty. Slowly move your thumb and index finger off cheeks, away from face toward windshield, and then up to the top of the car to help intensify the movement of the cheeks. Do this twice while on the way to an important meeting or a party. Your face will feel and look refreshed.

CAR EXERCISE #6: NOSE SHORTENER

Use the forefinger to push the tip of the nose up and hold firmly in place. Flex your nose down by pulling your upper lip down over the teeth and holding for a second before releasing the lip. Repeat thirty-five times, feeling the nose tip push against the finger each time. Remember to keep breathing at a steady rate as you work. This exercise stimulates blood circulation in your upper lip and nose and helps warm up the face.

CAR EXERCISE #7: MOUTH CORNER LIFT

Close your lips together. Tighten the corners of your mouth into hard clusters. Do not clench your teeth, and maintain steady breathing as you go. Lightly place your thumb and index finger on opposite corners of your mouth. Keep sucking in the corners of your mouth and *visualize* the corners turning up in a tiny smile and then turning down in a tiny frown. Pull thumb and index finger away from the corners of your mouth toward the windshield in small up-and-down motions to help you visualize the mouth corners at work. Push against the steering wheel with your other hand. Continue to "work" the corners of your mouth until you feel the burn. Hold the burn for a count of twenty, pulsing the thumb and index finger up and down.

CAR EXERCISE #8: LIP SHAPER

Press your upper and lower lips together. Imagine that you're crushing a pencil in the center of your lips. Put your index finger between your lips, in the center. While pressing the lips together, pull your finger slowly, toward the windshield, to lengthen the imaginary pencil. Push against the steering wheel with your other hand to intensify the resistance. Continue until you feel a burn in your upper lip, then pulse your finger up and down for a count of thirty.

CAR EXERCISE #9: NASAL LABIAL SMOOTHER

Pull your upper and lower lips away from each other to open your mouth into a long O. Pull your upper mouth corners up into a smile—using only your upper lip. Pull your nose up and wrinkle it like a rabbit while smiling with the upper lip. Forcefully push your upper lip down and keep it pressed against your teeth. You should feel the pull along the sides of your nose. Use your thumb and index finger to follow the energy up and down along the sides of your nose. Continue this movement until you feel the burning sensation along the nasal labial fold. Push away from the steering wheel. Hold the position and pulse the fingers up and down in the air quickly to intensify the burn for a count of twenty.

CAR EXERCISE #10: NECK STRENGTHENER

The unusual method involved in this exercise provides excellent neck strengthening and toning results. Grasp the front of your neck with one hand as if choking yourself. Push your chin out away from your body, then relax. Keep your other hand on the steering wheel and press against it for increased tension. Repeat this action thirty times, feeling your neck muscles flex under your fingers each time.

CAR EXERCISE #11: JAW STRENGTHENER

Open your mouth and roll your lower lip in tight over the lower teeth. Pull the corners of your mouth to the back and roll them in tightly. Keep your upper lip pressing down against your teeth. Open and close your jaw in a slow scooping motion, using the corners of your mouth to open and close, pulling the chin up a half inch with each scoop. *Imagine* scooping up chocolates with your jaw. *Visualize* the sides of your face lifting up. Move one hand up in front of the lower face as you imagine that the sides of your face are moving up through the top of the car. Push against the steering wheel for resistance with each scoop. When you are finished, the chin should be pointing toward the top of the car.

CAR EXERCISE #12: FACE WIDENER

Open your mouth and pull the corners to the back teeth. Roll in the corners of your mouth as hard as you can. Keep your upper lip against the upper teeth. *Visualize* big, apple-round cheeks growing out the corners of your mouth. Use the thumb and index finger of one hand to make small circles away from your face to help "pull" the energy out and fill in the gaunt area, while pushing away from the steering wheel with your other hand. Keep the corners of your mouth pulled back. Continue until you feel the muscles burn, making fast circles with the thumb and index finger to intensify the burn. Count to thirty.

CAR EXERCISE #13: FACE SLIMMER

Open your mouth and forcefully roll your lips over the teeth. Pull the corners of your mouth to the back teeth and roll them in tightly. *Visualize* the sides of your face moving up past the jawline. With fingers spread out, move one hand up the front of your face to help move the energy up along the sides of the face. Move the energy up until you feel the burn along the sides of your face. Push away from the steering wheel. Hold and count to thirty-five.

CAR EXERCISE #14: NECK AND CHIN TONER

Sit up straight, with your shoulders relaxed and your head held high. Close your lips and smile *only* with your upper lip. Place one hand at the base of the throat, over the collarbone, and pull down slightly on the skin with a firm grip. Tilt head back and release. You'll feel a strong pull on the chin and neck muscles. Tilt your head backward and forward to the original position thirty times.

6

YOUR SKIN CARE PROGRAM

I believe in a natural, self-disciplined approach to beauty, because it's the simplest and healthiest way for a woman to develop good habits and maintain her unique good looks. Doing Facercise regularly can help you gain a more youthful appearance, but this coupled with a daily, preventive skin care regimen is an even more effective beauty formula.

Practicing preventive skin care every day is absolutely vital if you want to maintain a glowing, youthful complexion. This holds true even if you're a teenager, for today's poor cleansing habits or failure to use sunscreen can lead to tomorrow's serious skin problems or wrinkles. Your skin is an external organ, and it's exposed every day of your life—no wonder it ages faster than any other organ.

Skin is highly vulnerable to various factors in the environment, especially the climate and air pollution. Internal environments also affect skin: if your emotional life is stormy, your face can look strained or tired. If you're under stress and not sleeping enough or eating properly, it will show on your face. Believe me, the skin requires regular attention and special nurturing throughout life to look its best.

A CRASH COURSE IN SKIN BASICS

The skin is composed of three layers: the epidermis, the dermis, and the subcutaneous tissue, also known as the fatty layer.

The outer layer of skin, or epidermis, consists of dead and dying cells which are constantly flaking off and being replaced with new ones arising from the base of the layer. New cells appear on the epidermis every twenty-eight to thirty days, but the cycle can be accelerated by conditions such as sunburn, windburn, poor sleeping habits, harsh cleansing, and skin irritations. Conditions such as these will affect the moisture balance in the epidermal cells and influence skin texture. The epidermis can be fed and nourished through careful skin cleansing, toning, and moisturizing.

Containing blood vessels, hair follicles, and nerves, the dermis layer is also home to collagen and elastin fibers, and two essential skin glands. These are the sebaceous and the sweat glands. The sebaceous glands secrete an oil called sebum. When this substance is produced in excess, the skin erupts in pimples. The sweat glands secrete water and salts. The oil and water created in the dermis form an emulsion that protects and lubricates the epidermis. This emulsion also prevents oil and moisture loss, thus helping normalize the acid (pH) balance of the skin.

Collagen and elastin diminish in production as we age. This causes the connective and supporting tissues in our skin to sag and become slack. Sagging combined with a lack of oil and moisture causes lines, furrows, and wrinkles. If the dermis is undernourished and has poor blood circulation, toxins may get stored in skin, causing the sebaceous glands to produce excess oil, which means eruptions on the epidermal layer. The condition of the dermis decisively shapes skin tone and contours.

The third and innermost layer is the subcutaneous tissue, which is the fatty yet firm foundation of the skin. Acting as an internal cushion, the subcutaneous layer protects organs and deep tissues from the bumps and blows of daily life while insulating against the loss of body heat.

We are all born with normal skin, but genetics and hormones—two factors beyond our control—determine our complexions as we get older. But you can improve the condition of your skin through a healthy, positive lifestyle, good nutrition, exercise, and dedicated skin care habits. Taking good care of your body and mind is the master key to looking good—and maintaining healthy skin.

The largest and most visible body organ, the skin is nourished by blood. Sleeping well, eating nutritious foods, and increasing the flow of blood to your outer skin tissues via exercise increases blood circulation and enhances the health of your skin.

As you know by now, the skin is shaped by bone structure and underlying muscle tissues. But it's also molded by the protein-based connective tissues containing collagen and elastin.

Collagen and elastin are fibrous strands that help make skin supple and plump. Have you ever seen a woman who's had collagen injections in her lips? These injections give the lips a full, "bee-stung" shape. Elastin helps connect and support the skin; its elastic qualities help create supple skin tone. A diminishing supply of collagen and elastin in aging skin is what causes it to sag. Collagen injections and implants are very costly, temporary treatments. Since collagen and elastin can never be naturally restored to aging skin, all exercise, and especially facial exercises, can help compensate by building up the underlying muscles, thus greatly improving the strength and beauty of your skin.

A literal bodyguard, your skin serves as a barrier against the sun's dangerous radiation, and filters out dirt and toxins in the air. Just as a full-length mirror reflects your health, your skin registers your living habits and what kind of beauty care you practice. Because what you put inside your body dramatically influences how your skin looks, let's begin with how and what you need to feed yourself to achieve a healthy complexion.

OXYGEN

Of course we need food and water to live, but from the moment we're born, we must breathe in oxygen from the air or we'll never survive. Apart from being the essential vehicle for the production of usable energy, oxygen is also the body's executive assistant. It works around the clock, helping synthesize fats, proteins, carbohydrates, and other substances in our food that help build and maintain cells, organs, muscles, bones—and all other bodily structures.

Having a good oxygen supply is an essential requirement for building a healthy body, mind, and of course, skin. Although some people use air purifiers in their home and office to improve the quality of the air they breathe, a mechanical purifier will never benefit your skin as much as regular exercise will. That's right, the most effective way to clear your skin through increased oxygen intake is to exercise at least three times a week. Perhaps you've noticed a healthy flush all over your skin after you've worked out—this glow is the result of increased blood circulation, a by-product of high oxygen intake.

Clinical research studies conducted in various countries have proven that regular aerobic exercise—exercise that involves elevating your heart and breathing rates to higher-than-average levels for twenty minutes or more, three times a week or more—keeps you healthier, more fit, and more relaxed.

Physical activity greatly benefits the skin by increasing the flow of blood throughout skin tissue, bringing oxygen and other nutrients needed for maintenance and repair of skin cells. Oxygenated blood helps process toxins and internal pollutants that damage skin and connective tissues. When you exercise hard enough to make your skin flush, you can see how blood is circulating vigorously throughout your body.

If you're not athletic, even mild exercise, such as twenty minutes of brisk daily walking, will help get your blood pumping and your complexion blooming. In either case, it's always wise to get your physician's approval before starting an exercise program.

Deep breathing is also a mild but effective form of aerobic exercise, and, like Facercise, you can do it anywhere. Even as you drive, sit at your desk, ride elevators, or do housework, deep breathing can make your body pump more blood everywhere, from your brain to your feet. Like an internal massage, deep yogic breathing gives you a calm but energized feeling.

Most of the time, we breathe shallowly, using only our upper lungs. Deep breathing means breathing from your diaphragm, which is in your stomach area.

Here's how you do deep breathing: Sit up straight with shoulders relaxed. Do not lean forward. Inhaling through your nose, slowly fill your lungs with a deep breath, beginning by expanding your stomach area as you inhale. Eventually, you should feel the air moving into the top of your lungs. When you've reached maximum breathing capacity, hold the breath for one second, then slowly exhale through your mouth. Relax and breathe normally for four breaths. Repeat this process ten times. Deep breathing is a healthful and effective way to elevate your energy and clear your skin. I urge you to practice this method whenever you can.

WATER

Your body needs water more than any other liquid. Drink eight or more glasses a day in addition to the other fluids you take in. This helps your body eliminate impurities, which leads to clearer skin. In addition, water helps reduce puffiness around the eyes and control hunger by making you feel fuller. Maintaining a healthy water balance is especially important for women. Drinking eight or more glasses of water a day can help you reduce premenstrual puffiness. Bottled mineral water contains less toxins than tap water and is thus better for you. Water carafes that contain renewable filters remove unpleasant taste and odor from the tap and are economical alternatives to drinking mineral water. Only reverse osmosis filters, however, remove chlorine and other impurities from water. Get one of these for your kitchen and you'll have a high-quality water supply.

DIET

Proper nutrition is a vital part of the Facercise program. We can't be eating an imbalanced diet, such as one high in fatty, salty, and sugary foods—and expect to have the strength and enthusiasm to work at changing our facial contours through Facercise. To build strong, supportive facial muscles with a fabulous clear complexion, plus slow down the aging process, you'll have to choose what you eat and drink with care. You *are* what you eat—and you'll look it!

We've all read and heard about various diets that are said to promote clear skin. But everybody's chemistry is different. The only way to learn what kind of vitamins and minerals your body (and skin) needs is to have a nutritionist take a blood sample and send it to a laboratory for a detailed analysis. Although it's impossible to recommend any one diet, there are a few skin-friendly guidelines to keep in mind when making food choices.

Eating a diet that's low in meats and cheese and high in fresh fruits, vegetables, and grains is a great way to feed your skin. Meats and cheeses are high in fat and protein and are difficult to digest. Animal products stimulate mucous production in the body, causing puffiness. On the other hand, the vitamins and minerals in fresh fruits and vegetables help build and repair cells. Many nutritional studies support the finding that vitamins such as C, E, and A, plus minerals like selenium and zinc, combat the breakdown of collagen and elastin, your skin's supporting and connective tissues.

When it comes to diet no-nos, salt is very high on the list. Salt makes you retain water and can make your face, and the rest of your body, look puffier. Never add salt to your food. Instead, use herbs and spices if you crave extra flavor. Remember that there is enough salt in a balanced diet to satisfy your body's requirements.

Because it promotes water retention, drinking alcohol is one of the surest ways to make your face look puffy. And apart from containing lots of calories, alcohol also dehydrates your skin. If you do drink, do so in moderation. And drink a glass of water for every alcoholic drink you imbibe. Water can help your body metabolize and excrete the alcohol more efficiently.

As for sugar, beware! Nutritionists know that eating sugary foods is the surest way to gain weight through empty calories. It is unclear whether sugar intake causes pimples, but it is clear that, although it initially gives you a rush, for twenty minutes or so, sugar is a depressant that can bring your energy level down. In the long run, the less sugar you consume, the more energy you'll have.

ANTI-AGING SUPPLEMENTS

As for anti-aging vitamin and mineral supplements, also known as antioxidants, there are many that have been clinically proven to protect the body from damaging free radicals. Free radicals are oxidants, or generators of toxic oxygen forms, that wage continual destructive sprees, causing molecular, cellular, and tissue damage. Although free radicals can also be beneficial, most of the time they act like internal saboteurs, attacking other cells and contributing to the development of various health problems and diseases. The effects of free radicals not only age the cells in your body— they also make your skin look old, gray, and lined.

Although free-radical activity occurs throughout our lives, these oxygen terrorists start doing serious damage when we're age forty and older. Free radicals are most often ingested in rancid food or through polluted air. Air pollutants include nitrogen oxides, ozone, and sulfur oxides. When inhaled, these substances generate free radicals.

If you smoke, or live with someone who does, realize that many of the toxic elements in cigarette smoke are oxidants. Smoking is one of the most damaging things you can do to your body and skin. This is because cigarette smoke contains high amounts of nitrogen oxides, which are themselves free radicals! When they get in the body, nitrogen oxides can react with polyunsaturated fatty acids inside cellular membranes, causing rancidification, rigidification, and death of cells. Clinical studies have shown, however, that vitamin E can help guard against these reactions.

Researchers established the cancer-causing potential of cigarette smoking decades ago. Many studies have concluded that free-radical activity is the primary cancer-causing factor in smoking. Nonsmokers can also be affected by the toxic terrorists in cigarette smoke. I know smoking is a difficult habit to give up, but you must try. Overwhelming scientific evidence shows that smoking is unhealthy.

The most widely used antioxidants include vitamins B12, E, C, and A, folic acid, and the trace mineral selenium. Beta-carotene and copper are also highly touted. Because everyone's biochemistry is unique, you should check with a nutritionist before going on an antioxidant supplement program. Most important, no pregnant woman should take any vitamin, mineral, or food supplement without first consulting her physician.

SLEEP

One of the most essential but most neglected ways to nourish skin is sound sleep habits. Human beings are governed by natural biological rhythms, called circadian rhythms. In other words, it is more natural for people to go to bed before midnight and wake in the early morning than it is for people to go to bed at three in the morning and rise at noon.

International studies show that an overwhelming number of people are sleep-deprived. Make the effort to keep a regular bedtime—say eleven o'clock—and get at least seven hours of sleep each night. Your whole body, especially your skin, will feel and look more alive.

YOUR SKIN CARE HABITS

Now that we've covered internal skin care, let's look at how you need to care for the outside. Careful cleansing is the first step in any proper skin care regimen. Dirt and dead skin cells need to be removed from the face in the morning and at night, possibly more if you exercise, have oily skin, or live in a polluted environment. Besides stimulating blood circulation in the face, thorough cleansing opens and cleanses pores. In addition, it helps prevent the skin's oils from clogging up and enlarging pores.

After cleansing comes moisturizing. After you cleanse in the morning, apply a moisturizer and then a sunscreen of at least SPF 30 to protect skin from ultraviolet radiation. (The sunscreen should be applied before makeup base.) The more you are exposed to the sun, the more your skin will age. A suntan is actually a sign of skin damage, and if you want to safeguard against wrinkles, *please* wear a sunscreen every day and stay out of the sun.

After cleansing at night, use a nightcream that will nourish and repair skin while you sleep. Eye creams are unnecessary if you're using a light but penetrating nightcream. The eye area lacks oil glands and the skin is extremely thin: heavy creams can actually weigh the skin down and promote wrinkles. Do yourself a favor and avoid rich, thick moisturizing eye creams.

No skin care regimen is complete without exfoliation, the clearing away of dead skin. Regular exfoliation with a botanically-based enzyme mask will get rid of the old and bring in the new. In my experience, the enzyme masks that work the best contain proteins, RNA, L-lysine, and proline. These cleanse and penetrate to tighten the epidermis. A good enzyme mask will constrict, tone, and tighten skin while drawing out impurities from the pores.

The skin care products that I find most valuable for all skin types are transdermal, meaning that they are so water soluble that they are actually stored in the skin for hours. Because they penetrate and rest inside the skin, transdermal preparations favorably influence the functions of cells and glands within the dermis. How to find high-quality transdermal products? Dermatologists and skin care salon estheticians are the most knowledgeable sources for these. You may, however, find some good ones on your own. Be sure to read labels and check for "transdermal" properties.

Although controversial, the vitamin A derivative retin-A does have its merits as an acne treatment. In the late 1980s, some researchers claimed that it could undo years of skin damage caused by aging and suntanning. I have never seen this happen. Rather, retin-A can smooth out fine surface lines—but that's about all. In addition, no one knows what the long-term positive or negative effects of this cosmetic pharmaceutical may be.

I have used various skin care products containing alpha hydroxy acids, and many dermatologists and estheticians recommend these for their superior cleansing and skin-balancing properties.

Some cosmetic manufacturers claim that new, oxygen-bearing emulsions can actually penetrate the skin and bring other nutrients, such as vitamins A and E, directly into skin cells for repair work. Remember the previous discussion of oxygen, the great vehicle for producing energy in the body? Oxygen-bearing cosmetics are some of the most highly touted products on today's market. The main active ingredient in oxygen cosmetics is medical-grade hydrogen peroxide. While no clinical evidence exists to confirm these manufacturer's claims, it's a fact that bacteria, which contributes to skin problems such as acne, cannot survive in an oxygen-rich environment. This strongly suggests that oxygen acts as an antibacterial agent on or in the skin.

One oxygen cosmetic that I often use happens to be drugstore hydrogen peroxide. You can experiment on your own with oxygen-based treat-ments by pouring a bottle of hydrogen peroxide into a plastic spray bottle. Spritz it on your face in the morning and you'll feel and look refreshed. I pour a whole eight-ounce bottle of it in the bath after a long day, and I feel as if I've had a full body facial. (A hydrogen peroxide bath is also a great remedy for jet lag.) Steam baths are another low-tech yet effective method for opening pores and cleansing skin.

BODY SKIN SECRETS

Although I use moisturizers on my face, I take a different view of how to nourish the skin on the rest of my body. It may sound sacrilegious from a skin care expert, but the best way to achieve soft, supple skin is to never use moisturizers on your body. I know I don't. Here's what I do instead: every morning, before I take a shower or bath, I give myself a quick "body facial" that hails from Baden Baden, one of Europe's oldest and most renowned spas.

Use a *dry* sisal or loofah with mitts for both hands that are connected by a strap. Put a hand in the mitts and start on the sole of your foot, making counterclockwise circular motions—this stimulates blood flow in the di-rection of your heart. Circle up your leg to your stomach, then make circular motions on the top of your free hand and up the arm and over the chest area. Change mitt to other hand and start on the other foot, repeating the pattern. Then put both your hands in mitts and shimmy the scrubbing fibers up the back of your legs, buttocks, back, and neck. Rinse the fibers in water once a week and let dry overnight.

By stimulating blood circulation and sloughing off dead skin cells, this daily treatment energizes you and helps eliminate toxins from the skin. Dry exfoliation promotes a healthy, pink glow and soft, fresh-feeling skin. Another benefit is that it's cost-effective and can save you the expense of body lotion. A good quality loofah or sisal lasts several months.

NIGHTTIME SKIN CARE SECRETS

Some people barely recognize themselves when they get up in the morn-ing. This is because they sleep on their stomachs with their heads pushed into the pillow and they wake up with puffy areas and sleep lines that make them look tired and creased. You can avoid this situation by conditioning yourself to sleep only on your back, without a pillow under your head.

Instead, use a neck roll and put the pillow under your knees before going to sleep. You'll see the difference in the morning.

As I explained earlier, we move our faces in sleep the same way that we do during waking hours. You frown and smile often during the day; you repeat these same expressions as you dream. To reduce lines in the forehead or between the eyebrows, apply surgical tape on skin furrows before going to bed. Try it for four nights in a row and you'll see that your skin looks smoother in the morning. I routinely tape the area between my eyebrows before going to bed, as this helps smooth out the lines.

Let's face it: the only thing standing between you and beautiful skin is your mind. If you can visualize how your eating, lifestyle, and grooming habits will affect your looks, then you will behave carefully and achieve your beauty goals. Every method and tip I discussed in this chapter can be easily integrated into your daily life. I encourage you to keep Facercising and remember to pamper your skin every day, morning and night.

In the eleven years I've been teaching Facercise, I've seen people of all ages and walks of life enjoy remarkable and healthy changes after devoting twenty minutes of their day to the program. Whenever you need encouragement, take another look at Chapter Three's dramatic before and after photos. I've also included on the following pages some actual letters of testimony and thanks I've received from clients over the years. I promise you that by doing the exercises in this book, you, too, can give yourself a natural face-lift.

Facercise has taken me around the world to teach people how to realize their inner and outer beauty. Do you know the old Chinese saying "When the student is ready, the Master appears"? Well, experience has taught me that many people on this planet are ready for Facercise. When I train people and see how their faces change after doing the program, I feel great satisfaction and happiness for them. Why? Because they did it themselves, and they feel and look terrific.

You, too, can revitalize your own unique beauty. If you want a more youthful and toned-looking face, a rosier complexion, firmer skin, and sparkling eyes, believe me, all you have to do is Facercise.

IN THEIR OWN WORDS

Letters from Facercisers

Dear Carole,

I'm writing you this letter on my 50th birthday to tell you how much enjoyment I have already received from my "big gift," Facercise. Although it's only been four weeks since I completed my classes with you, my husband and family are thrilled with the results. My husband feels it's the best money he has ever spent on a present. I feel great and all my friends think I look years younger. The best part is that there was no doctor, no cutting, and no waiting months for it to "relax." My results were almost instant. Thanks for the new me.

> Warmest regards,
> *Jane Miller*
> *Scottsdale, AZ*

Dear Carole,

My face is looking better every day! A friend asked me, after only *two weeks*, what I was doing to it. I can't believe how quickly it worked. The bags under my eyes have disappeared and I have developed great new cheek-bones. Many thanks once again for your help and inspiration.

> Yours sincerely,
> *K.M.*
> *London, England*

Dear Carole,

When I signed up for your course of facial exercise, I was skeptical. It has now been twelve days and I have had at least six clients and friends ask me what I was doing for my face because I really looked good.

I now have cheeks, larger lips and a wider face, something I thought was impossible with my features! I also have a problem with TMJ, and I have noticed that the jaw exercises have helped relieve my pain and tension. Your program is unbelievable and I can't thank you enough. It has really helped my confidence!

Best wishes,
Joan M. Lessner
Redondo Beach, CA

Dear Carole,

After eye surgery several years ago, I trained with you and your program and was pleasantly surprised to find my eyes wider and my face much stronger. Had I known prior to my surgery what your program could do for me, I would have never undergone the surgery. I'm confident in saying to everyone that they should train the muscles in their face. This training has given me more confidence and personal satisfaction in my appearance.

Love,
Jan Fuson
Redondo Beach, CA

Thanks to Facercise and Carole Maggio I feel like a new woman!

Facercise is absolutely fabulous! I love the one-to-one training with Carole: she has introduced me to a new world of extensive facial exercises which have now become a part of my daily routine. In only twenty minutes, whether I exercise at home or in the car, I feel refreshed and invigorated, knowing the results are truly rewarding.

I started the exercises a month ago and already have had many, many wonderful compliments on how I look. It had been a while since I had seen some of my friends and when we were recently together at a convention, they commented on how great and "different" I look. The "difference" is due, of course, to my facial exercises.

When working with Carole during the face training, she took a photograph of me at the beginning, the middle, and the end of the sessions. What can I say? The pictures said it all! The visible changes are absolutely remarkable, and all in just five days!

Facercise has definitely made me feel younger and more attractive. Thank you, Carole, and I LOVE YOU *FACERCISE!*

Alexa Coon
Washington, DC

Dear Carole,

I want to tell you how my progress has been since I took the Facercise course about three years ago. Remember, I came to you really out of desperation, as I had exhausted all other obvious options. I wanted to get rid of my acute scarring and had had three dermabrasions already. My only other option, according to several plastic surgeons, was a face-lift, which most likely would have to be done every couple of years. Well, my results with Facercise have been beyond what I had hoped for.

My eyes, which were always half-closed, are more open and brighter. My acute scarring is barely visible because I've been able to pump my cheek area out. I always had pale, yellow, lifeless skin; my skin is now pink and much brighter. My husband, a medical doctor, was kind of doubtful about the course, but he was astonished by the results and has given me nothing but encouragement to share this with others.

Love,
Laurie Ellen McGarry
Carmel, CA

Dear Carole,

My mother taught me to write thank-you letters, but this is the first I have ever written for "services rendered," and yet it is probably the most heart-felt of any.

As you may remember, I was quite skeptical of the value of face exercises when I read the article about you in *Longevity* and called you with a thousand questions; however, I was desperate for help and mortally afraid of surgery, not to mention that the cost was way beyond my means. It was talking to three of your satisfied clients that finally convinced me to take the training.

Yes, I know, Carole, I was a difficult student; but you, against heavy odds, created a remarkable change in my face—well, really I should say you helped *me* create the change which makes me very proud of myself.

What brought me to the point of writing this thank-you letter was my seeing my college roommate last week at a Pan Hellenic luncheon, and knowing me so well and feeling she could say anything at all to me no matter how outrageous, she popped out with, "My God, Nancy, who did your facelift? You look fabulous!" Wow, what a testimony to what you and I achieved together!

Thank you, Carole,
Nancy Cooksey
Monterey, CA

Dear Ms. Maggio,

You asked for an update of my physical progress after my sessions doing Facercise. I am happy to report that the feeling has returned to my face, especially the right side. In addition, my face is fuller and the flatness has disappeared, just as you said it would.

My partner Paul is delighted with my progress; he was by my side during my long and painful ordeal with Bell's Palsy. Now he would like to schedule time with you.

Thank you for the healing and
uplifting program you've
developed,
George T.
Chicago, IL

Dear Carole,

I find myself at a loss for words to describe how I feel about your Facercise program, as I'm quite certain your many clients are. So here goes! THANK YOU! THANK YOU! THANK YOU! You have a magical gift in the Facercise Program.

Six days ago I began the facial exercises. Many of my friends have had plastic surgery; some, to my horror, look as though they are wearing a tight mask. Their faces look different to me, not better. A close personal friend has no feeling in her left cheek—the surgeon says it may return in time.

I am a woman in my sixties and thought my only option was to take my chances and go under the knife. I heard about you and, because of my fears, not because I believed a facial exercise program would work, I came to you.

You are remarkable. My face looks youthful again, and the sag in my jaw and neck is improving. Just this morning as I was leaving the gym, two women asked me what I had done to my face—I looked much younger and radiant to them.

To think that six days ago I felt hopeless and even depressed when I applied my makeup. I thank God for you, Carole Maggio, and will send clients to you. I now am planning a trip to London with the $10,000 I saved by choosing you instead of the surgeon.

Sincerely,
Anne Bennett
Palos Verdes, CA

PERSONAL CALENDAR

Here is a Facercise agenda that you can use to keep track of your exercises in that crucial first month—and in the months beyond. Remember to do all of the exercises twice a day, or more, depending on your goals.

#1. EYE ENHANCER

#2. LOWER EYELID STRENGTHENER

#3. FOREHEAD LIFT

#4. CHEEK DEVELOPER

#5. FACE ENERGIZER

#6. NOSE SHORTENER

#7. MOUTH CORNER LIFT

#8. LIP SHAPER

#9. NASAL LABIAL SMOOTHER

#10. NECK STRENGTHENER

#11. JAW STRENGTHENER

#12. FACE WIDENER

#13. FACE SLIMMER

#14. NECK AND CHIN TONER

1	2	3	4	5	6	7
Facercised all 14 exercises ___ times	Facercised all 14 exercises ___ times	Facercised all 14 exercises ___ times	Facercised all 14 exercises ___ times	Facercised all 14 exercises ___ times	Facercised all 14 exercises ___ times	Facercised all 14 exercises ___ times
8	9	10	11	12	13	14
Facercised all 14 exercises ___ times	Facercised all 14 exercises ___ times	Facercised all 14 exercises ___ times	Facercised all 14 exercises ___ times	Facercised all 14 exercises ___ times	Facercised all 14 exercises ___ times	Facercised all 14 exercises ___ times
15	16	17	18	19	20	21
Facercised all 14 exercises ___ times	Facercised all 14 exercises ___ times	Facercised all 14 exercises ___ times	Facercised all 14 exercises ___ times	Facercised all 14 exercises ___ times	Facercised all 14 exercises ___ times	Facercised all 14 exercises ___ times
22	23	24	25	26	27	28
Facercised all 14 exercises ___ times	Facercised all 14 exercises ___ times	Facercised all 14 exercises ___ times	Facercised all 14 exercises ___ times	Facercised all 14 exercises ___ times	Facercised all 14 exercises ___ times	Facercised all 14 exercises ___ times
29	30	31				
Facercised all 14 exercises ___ times	Facercised all 14 exercises ___ times	Facercised all 14 exercises ___ times				

ABOUT THE AUTHOR

Carole Maggio is a skin care specialist who for eleven years has taught Facercise to clients across the United States, Europe, the Middle East, and Japan. She has conducted beauty seminars at the University of London, served as instructor at one of Tokyo's foremost beauty establishments, and has lectured at conferences and before selected audiences around the world. She currently lives in Redondo Beach, California.